EIGHT INTENTIONS FOR SELF-HEALING

EIGHT INTENTIONS FOR SELF-HEALING

A PRACTICAL GUIDE TO RECLAIMING YOUR PERSONAL POWER

CAROLYN PITTS

INTEND WELL LLC

Copyright © 2025 by Carolyn Pitts

All rights reserved.

No part of this book may be reproduced in any form or by any electronic or mechanical means, including information storage and retrieval systems, without written permission from the author, except for the use of brief quotations in a book review.

The information given in this book should not be treated as a substitute for professional medical advice; always consult a medical practitioner. The author of this book does not dispense medical advice or prescribe the use of any technique as a form of treatment for physical, emotional, or medical problems. The intent of the author is only to offer information of a general nature to help you in your quest for emotional and spiritual well-being. In the event that you use any of the information in this book for yourself, which is your right, the author and publisher assume no responsibility for your actions. Neither the author nor the publisher can be held responsible for any loss, claim, or damage arising out of the use, or misuse, of the suggestions made, the failure to take medical advice, or for any other material on third-party websites.

Links to information provided by third-party websites were correct at the time of publication.

Library of Congress Control Number: 2025912779

Digital ISBN: 979-8-9927655-0-2

Paperback ISBN: 979-8-9927655-1-9

Audio ISBN: 979-8-9927655-2-6

To preserve the privacy of individuals involved, names and certain identifying details have been changed. Some of the characters described are composites.

CONTENTS

PART 1
WELCOME
1. All Healing is Self-Healing — 3
2. Ready, Set, Go! — 7

PART 2
MEET THE EIGHT INTENTIONS
3. The Demonstrated Power of Intention — 25
4. Intentional Resilience — 29
5. Intentional Vibes — 45
6. Intentional Focus — 71
7. Intentional Mindset — 93
8. Intentional Release — 113
9. Intentional Nutrition — 135
10. Intentional Movement — 157
11. Intentional Relationships — 177
12. Living the Eight Intentions — 195

PART 3
SELF-EXPLORATION
13. Worksheets and Exercises — 201
   Chronic Anxiety Self-Assessment Tool — 203
   Chronic Anxiety Self-Assessment Tracker — 209
   Technique Practice Tracker — 211
   Mindset Map Exercise — 215
   Limiting Beliefs Exercise — 223
   Affirmations Exercise — 225
   Daily Food Diary Exercise — 229
   Daily Produce Tracker — 233
   Intentional Movement Practice Tracker — 235
   Mind the Gap Exercise — 237
   The Intend Well Wheel — 239

Notes — 245
Acknowledgments — 251
About the Author — 253

PART 1
WELCOME

ONE

ALL HEALING IS SELF-HEALING

ALL HEALING IS SELF-HEALING. Our bodies have the remarkable ability to defeat viruses, repair a sprained ligament, or grow new skin to close a cut.

In the case of serious injury or disease, our healing capacity benefits from the boost provided by the marvels of modern medicine. Yet if the cure were purely in the treatment, aspirin would ease every pain, antibiotics would defeat every infection, and chemotherapy would shrink every tumor. Medical professionals and pharmaceutical companies could offer money-back guarantees.

Ultimately, the effectiveness of any medical treatment relies on the robustness of our self-healing power. According to widely cited analysis, professional health care accounts for less than 20 percent of health outcomes.[1] [2] Yet, burdened by the stressors of modern daily living, we forget that the key to our vibrancy lies within us.

Compared to countries in Europe, Americans live shorter lives despite spending more on health care. Life expectancy in the United States was 78.4 years at birth in 2023, versus 82.5 years in comparable countries including Australia, Canada, and Europe. At the same time, health care costs in the United States continue to climb at an accelerating rate. In 2024, the Kaiser Family Foundation reported that one out of every five dollars goes to pay for health care.[3] In 1960, the rate was one out of every twenty dollars.

Chronic stress is implicated in several health challenges. Conditions including cancer, cardiovascular diseases (high blood pressure, heart disease), metabolic disorders (obesity, Type 2 diabetes), neurodegenerative diseases (Alzheimer's and Parkinson's), and gastrointestinal problems (ulcers, reflux, irritable bowel syndrome) improve when anxiety is reduced.

For the most part, these conditions do not bring on sudden death. Instead, they deliver a slow decline in vitality as standing for long periods, climbing stairs, remembering people's names, and carrying groceries become increasingly more difficult.

Our society shrugs off these challenges as bad genes or the inevitable result of aging, yet epigenetic research and studies of centenarians disprove such notions. It's no secret that nutritious foods, quality sleep, physical activity, and resilience to stress are important for optimal health. Instead of outsourcing our well-being to an overburdened healthcare system, we can reclaim our personal power to heal through intentional lifestyle choices.

If you are like me, some part of each day happens automatically, without your conscious awareness. My morning and bedtime routines are so familiar that my body goes through the motions all on its own.

For example, I brush my teeth every morning regardless of whether I feel like it or not. I don't engage in an internal debate about whether dental hygiene is necessary or consider the consequences of skipping a day. I just do it. What are some of the daily tasks that you do on autopilot?

The key to reclaiming our self-healing power is to first identify a lifestyle change that is appropriate for us and then integrate that activity into our daily routine. Experimentation may be necessary to find the best insertion point, but then the change becomes a habit with practice.

Five years ago, I started practicing yoga after I brush my teeth in the morning. In a few weeks, my daily yoga practice became automatic. Many mornings my mind whines in protest—*I don't feel like practicing yoga today*—but my body rolls out the mat anyway.

What works for me is not right for everyone, however. Because a one-size-fits-all approach is unrealistic, I offer flexible strategies to implement lifestyle changes in ways that are appropriate for you. Part 3 of this book ("Self-Exploration") is loaded with exercises and worksheets to support your unique path to self-healing power.

BEFORE WE JUMP IN, allow me to tell you about myself. For nearly thirty years, I have maintained certification as a Health Coach through the American Council on Exercise (ACE), which requires me to recertify every two years by demonstrating competence in the latest nutrition and lifestyle science.

My eagerness to help clients implement permanent improvements led me to expand my certification to include specializations in Behavior Change and Plant-Based Coaching. But this book is about so much more than the conventional diet and exercise advice.

What makes my approach unique is the emphasis on the biofield—the scientifically recognized energy field that surrounds and influences the body. I lean into my experience as a Healing Touch Professional to offer novel approaches to self-healing that are easy to learn, take minimal time to perform, and are highly effective.

These techniques are rooted in ancient wisdom that humans relied on for centuries before pharmaceuticals and surgery became the primary tools of medical treatment. While it may seem woo-woo at first, there is a plethora of scientific research that backs energy healing—some of which I will share with you.

Whether you are struggling with a chronic condition now or want to avoid debilitating disease in the future, you are the captain of your wellness, and this book is your map.

The information in these pages is just the beginning. I've also created a free online companion to make it easier for you to practice the techniques, set your own goals, and track your individual progress.

Scan the QR code below or visit CarolynPitts.com/eightintentions for instructional videos and full-size downloadable worksheets.

TWO
READY, SET, GO!

As I step into the shower, my brain starts cranking out a mental to-do list for the day ahead. Topping today's list is that smoldering issue at work that threatens to erupt into flames if I don't throw some water on it soon. As I reach for the nearly empty bottle of shampoo, I add it to my mental shopping list for Saturday…again. I hope I will remember to buy it this time. What else? I conjure a mental image of my planner, opened to today's date. It's Thursday, so that means back-to-back meetings. Oh no! I realize that status reports are due tomorrow. "Hurry up!" my inner voice admonishes. "You need to get to work early enough to tackle at least one of those before your first meeting."

Instantly, adrenaline and cortisol flood my bloodstream. On the outside, I look like a woman getting ready for work. But inside, I'm a heaving sea of churning thoughts and emotions. Shifting my anxiety level into overdrive is how I "power up" in the morning. Being steeped in urgency feels normal.

After a long day, I stay at work to knock out the remaining status reports while devouring a meal replacement bar from the stash in my desk drawer. At six-thirty in the evening, I head home to pick up my daughter for tonight's Girl Scout meeting. The troop is going camping in a few weeks. My mind is simultaneously planning meals for this camping trip while trying to remember exactly what I needed from the grocery store this morning but forgot to write down. Lost in thought, I run a red light. Screeching brakes and a blaring horn alert me to my near miss. Finally home at nine, I'm grouchy with hunger and oozing pent-up irritation from my day.

Walking in the door relieves me of the expectation to maintain professionalism throughout my long day. I snap at my husband and kids, surrendering my emotional self-control in a phenomenon known as "restraint collapse." Straining under the weight of a never-ending task list means that investing energy in relationships with my loved ones feels like one more obligation.

My anxiety left me feeling profoundly lonely; a stressed-out mind tends to imagine threats everywhere, forcing us to withdraw inside our emotional castle walls and raise the drawbridge. My body suffered from what I now know were symptoms of chronic anxiety: weight gain, headaches, irritable bowels, rigid shoulder muscles, and poor sleep.

Anxious people are short-tempered and overly critical, and they radiate a disconcerting nervous buzz like a hive of angry bees. I was desperate to change but didn't know how. I taped an index card with the word "Calm" in a lovely blue script to my computer monitor. It's no surprise that willing myself into calmness didn't work—but I didn't know what else to do.

THAT WAS THEN. Now, as I step into the shower, I feel a rush of gratitude that hot water is available with the twist of a knob. I lift the shampoo bottle to my nose, deeply inhaling the floral aroma. Before stepping out of the shower, I twist the knob to cold and laugh at the pleasing sensation of the icy water. I smile at my reflection in the bathroom mirror, whispering, "Hello, beautiful! I love you." My inner voice is much more polite these days. She knows that if she starts whining, I will shush her. Mistakes don't upset me like they used to. Instead, I chuckle, recalling how I used to aspire to unrealistic expectations. This is not to say that I am immune to stress. Life can still trigger a rush of adrenaline and cortisol, but the effect is short-lived, as I can quickly restore my sense of calmness. I've lost twenty pounds, stopped taking pain relievers, and found the restorative sleep I craved.

So, what happened? My transition started when I began studying Healing Touch (HT). Similar to Reiki or acupuncture, Healing Touch is a form of energy medicine that facilitates healing by grounding, centering, and balancing our electromagnetic aspects. (You will learn what that means in future chapters!) HT entered my life when I was eager to escape my cage of irritability. When I registered for HT training, I expected to learn how to heal other people—but the first person I healed was myself.

My HT instructors emphasized the importance of self-care, because healers can better serve our clients when we take care of ourselves first. I used HT to self-heal headaches, my cranky knees, and my chronic anxiety. These techniques are so simple anyone can learn them. We can teach them to our children before they have even developed the capacity to read.

As my stress level decreased, my exploration of self-healing expanded. I learned to make peace with my inner critic, conquer my perfectionism, and tune into my intuition. Intentional self-care created the calm new me who is lean, flexible, energetic, and sees the doctor only once a year for check-ups. Unlike many other people in their mid-sixties, I am not popping prescriptions or bemoaning the deterioration of health mistakenly associated with aging.

This book is the guide I needed when I taped the word "Calm" to my computer in a vain attempt to dispel my chronic anxiety. I've organized what I call my "energetic self-care routine" into eight intentions. Within the framework of these eight intentions, I will teach you practical techniques to help you reclaim your calm when life knocks you sideways.

Just as we wash the grime from our skin and brush food particles from between our teeth every day, these techniques work best when practiced regularly—not just when we feel stressed. So, I will also show you how to make self-healing part of your existing daily routine.

Here are some clues that this book is right for you.

Your health needs healing. Does the story of the stressed-out old me sound familiar? Do you suffer from chronic pain and irritability? Are you eager to discover the happier, healthier you but not sure how to start? In my situation, chronic anxiety was the root of my health complaints, but I didn't recognize the symptoms. Turn to the Chronic Anxiety Self-Assessment in the back of this book. If the list of symptoms looks familiar, you are in the right place.

You feel like you've tried everything. Stress interferes with our ability to understand and use new information. So, ironically, we can read an insightful book on personal growth but struggle to apply the wisdom to our personal situation. This book is filled with short, simple techniques to prepare the mind for learning.

You are ready to take action. Mental and emotional readiness is a prerequisite for any personal growth journey. If you have tried unsuccessfully to improve your health in the past, it may be that you were not adequately prepared. In the next section, you will find some questions to help you assess your readiness to make actionable changes in your life.

You are open to a holistic approach. Conventional healing approaches focus myopically on the physical body. As we will discover, optimum health requires a whole-body perspective—body, mind, and spirit.

You are committed to reclaiming your personal power to heal. No one learns to play the piano by reading a book about Chopin. Reclaiming your personal power to heal requires intentional effort. Are you willing to set aside excuses, stop arguing for your limitations, and make meaningful changes?

Throughout this book, I will ask you introspective questions designed to strengthen your self-awareness. To get the most out of the book, I encourage you to document your responses in writing using a separate journal or the printable worksheets in the book's online companion.

Tonya's Story

When we met for our first healing session, Tonya's primary concern was chronic pain from hip replacement surgery. Despite multiple rounds of physical therapy, she still walked unsteadily, relying on a cane for balance.

Tonya fell into such a deep, sonorous sleep during our third session that putting my hand on her shoulder and calling her name failed to rouse her. This happens often during an HT session. I see it as an indication that deep healing is happening, so I wait until the client wakes up on their own.

Forty minutes later, Tonya opened her eyes. The transformation was noticeable—she looked lighter, brighter, and more alert. Tonya said she was amazed by how good she felt. She got off the table unaided and walked without pain. We closed the session by identifying actions that Tonya would take to sustain her continued self-healing.

When I saw Tonya a few weeks later, she was shuffling along with her cane again. As I soon discovered, Tonya had not followed through with her action plan from the previous session. Her commitment to her healing did not extend beyond coming to me for HT sessions.

Tonya's story is not uncommon. Too often, we focus on treatments instead of lifestyle changes. Perhaps you know someone who is searching for healing from outer sources instead of activating the power within themselves.

Assessing Your Readiness for Change

In my early days as a coach and healer, I mistakenly believed that my clients' progress depended on the adequacy of my abilities, so I felt responsible when their health issues persisted. But then I learned that I can't heal anyone—that, at its core, all healing is self-healing. Reclaiming our personal power requires a significant personal investment of energy and persistence.

As an ACE Behavior Change Specialist, I understand that this is easier said than done. Change can be extremely difficult even in life-threatening situations. Between 50 and 80 percent of patients with chronic illnesses struggle to implement and maintain healthy behaviors.[1] If you have tried and failed repeatedly to improve your health in the past, rest assured that change is still possible.

Sometimes, we embark on a health improvement journey before we are ready. Perhaps our doctor has warned us to stop smoking, or our spouse nags us to lose weight, but—like Tonya — our motivation is lackluster. Perhaps we are afraid we might fail. Perhaps we are constrained by limiting beliefs. Or perhaps we underestimate the commitment required for meaningful and lasting transformation.

The difference between those who achieve their wellness goals and those who don't is their readiness for change. Evaluating our mental and emotional readiness increases the probability of success any time we tackle a new goal.

Are you ready to reclaim your self-healing power? Here are some questions to help you assess your readiness.

To get the most out of this assessment, I highly recommend answering these questions in writing. The act of moving your hand across a page slows your thoughts, allowing unexpected insights to emerge, like sunlight breaking free of the clouds after a storm. Grab your journal or some blank sheets of paper, and let's dive in.

Know Your Whys

Change happens when the perceived pain of staying as we are outweighs the perceived pain of doing things differently. Just knowing that something is good for us may not be enough to keep us going when inevitable setbacks occur. Health goals that someone else goaded us into setting are too flimsy to withstand the headwinds of our biological resistance to change. On the other hand, strong internal motivation is the wind beneath our wings when we feel tempted to give up.

In the past, I tried and failed to resist sugary treats, forgo my nightly glass of wine, and kick my caffeine habit…until I found a reason powerful enough to sustain my commitment. In each case, scientific research convinced me that the cost to my health outweighed the pleasure I derived from consuming things that weren't good for me.

- Why do you want to improve your health?
- Is it because your doctor or a loved one suggested that your health needs improving? Or are you driven by internal motivation?
- Are your whys shining brightly enough to illuminate the path to a calmer, healthier, future you?

Know Your Why Nots

When we undertake positive changes in our life, there can be unexpected tradeoffs. For example, a gamer who decides to spend less time online may miss socializing virtually with their gamer friends. The desire to stop drinking alcohol may lead to foregoing happy-hour get-togethers with colleagues after work.

A smoker may worry about gaining weight if she gives up cigarettes.

Recall that imbibing an adrenaline-cortisol cocktail was how I used to "power up" in the morning. A why not for conquering my anxiety was that I credited my career success to my chronic urgency. I had to release the belief that my productivity depended on self-imposed stress.

Although I didn't know it at the time, my client Tonya had a why not for reclaiming her self-healing capability. Her lengthy recovery from hip replacement surgery prevented her from returning to a job that she hated.

- What motivation do you have to ignore the greener grass and stay where you are?
- Imagine your future self smiling, peaceful, handling life's difficulties with ease. When we pick up one end of a stick, the other end comes with it. As you pick up the stick of wellness, what undesirable consequences might be attached to it?

Know Your Sacrifices

Before marriage and kids, I had the freedom to work out at the gym a few times a week. The other regulars and I dreaded January, as the parking lot, locker room, and aerobics classes were packed with newbies, but we knew the crowds would thin by February. Sales of gym memberships soar in January because excitement about the New Year is mistaken as readiness for change. It takes just a few clicks of the mouse to buy a gym membership, but putting on our workout clothes, getting to the gym, exercising, and showering afterward can be a two-hour commitment every time we go. The newbies' failure to allocate the time required to use their gym memberships is a big reason the crowd size was back to normal in four weeks.

Change requires sacrifice. To add a new activity to our

routine, we have to make space by swapping out an existing activity. For example, I sacrificed volunteering and social activities to write this book.

- What existing activities will you sacrifice to create space for change?
- Will those sacrifices free up enough time to read the chapters, practice the techniques, assess your progress, and reflect on your experience?

Know Your When

The hit song "Tomorrow" from the Broadway musical Annie brims with optimism about the future. Although today may be gray and lonely, the lyrics promise that tomorrow will be bright with sunshine. Yet—as the song reminds us—the irony is that tomorrow never comes; it is always a day away.

- Are you ready to begin transformational change now?
- If not now, then put a start date on your calendar. Some people start their change journey on the first day of the month or their birthday. Perhaps you want to start when you finish that big project at work.
- If you won't be ready to start within the next two weeks, what conditions need to be met for you to feel ready? Why are those conditions important?

Don't wait for everything to be perfectly aligned because— just like tomorrow— that time will never come. Imperfect progress is better than no progress at all.

Know Your Who

Your wellness journey impacts the people in your life. Your relationships with your romantic partner, children, friends, and coworkers will improve as you become more calm and joyful within yourself. Consider how the people in your life can support you in your journey. Perhaps the coworkers you eat lunch with will understand if you want to dine alone some days so you can read while you eat. Perhaps you and a friend could serve as each other's accountability partner as you explore this book together.

- Who are your allies?
- How will you recruit their support?

On the flip side, consider whether anyone in your life would prefer for you to stay as you are. The dynamics of a relationship can be disrupted when one person starts to change while the other would prefer they remain the same. For example, my neighbor's marriage ended when she conquered chronic obesity.

- Is there anyone who might sabotage your self-improvement plan?
- What can you do to mitigate their resistance to your change?
- How will you stay on track over their objections?

Finally, look inside. Years ago, I received a promotion at work that entitled me to a private office with a view of downtown. Back then I had never heard of imposter syndrome, so I didn't recognize the symptoms. Every morning when I walked into my new office, I thought to myself, "I can't believe I have my own office!" If we don't believe that we deserve something, chances are that we won't keep it. Sure enough, I lost my position—and my office—in the next reorganization.

- Accomplishing your health goals will change how you see yourself as well as how other people see you. Are you prepared to embrace your new identity?

- Have you engaged in self-sabotage in the past? If so, do you believe that you deserve personal growth now?

Know Your Superpower

We all have strengths. Sometimes, we overlook our superpowers because they come so naturally to us that we assume they're easy for everyone.

It is natural for me to stick with a project until it is complete. I don't start a new book until I finish the one I am reading, or cast on a new knitting project until I bind off the one on my needles. It wasn't until a friend mentioned all her half-finished endeavors that I saw my stick-to-it-iveness as a superpower.

- What activities confound others but are effortless for you? Perhaps you excel at organizing events, solving puzzles, or devouring a book in record time.
- What has worked well for you in past efforts to improve your health?
- How will your superpowers support you?

Know Your Kryptonite

Just as Superman's strength crumbled in the presence of kryptonite, we all face challenges that diminish our capability. Perfectionism was core to my identity for most of my adult life. While initially proud of my attention to detail, I eventually realized it was a liability. My colleagues were able to shrug off their mistakes without consequence; why couldn't I? Late in life, I realized that deep-seated insecurity fed my fear of mistakes. As my self-worth increased, I learned to forgive my shortcomings, although a tiny piece of me still cringes—just for a moment—when I screw up.

- What is your kryptonite that holds you back from living the life you deserve?
- Think back to unsuccessful attempts to improve your wellness in the past. What got in the way of your success? Perhaps you underestimated the time commitment, or your heart wasn't really in it. Perhaps you let the first slip derail your intention because you didn't have confidence in your ability.
- What will you do differently this time?

Now it's time to reflect on your readiness to move forward. Referring back to your written answers to the questions in this section, answer yes or no to each statement in the Readiness Self-Assessment table.

Readiness Self-Assessment

	Yes	No
I Know My Why *My reasons for making changes are powerful enough to sustain me through obstacles and setbacks.*	☐	☐
I Know My Why Not *The trade-offs from making changes to improve my self-healing are worth it.*	☐	☐
I Know My Sacrifices *I can allocate sufficient time to read the book and practice the techniques.*	☐	☐
I Know My When *I am ready to start within the next two weeks.*	☐	☐
I Know My Who *I believe that I deserve a better future, and I have a plan for engaging support from family, friends, and co-workers.*	☐	☐
I Know My Superpower *I can tap into my strengths to support my change.*	☐	☐
I Know My Kryptonite *I know what can sabotage my success, and I have a plan to mitigate it.*	☐	☐

How do you feel as you review your responses above? Clues that you are ready to move forward include:

- Most of the checkmarks are in the "yes" column, and the "no" items feel manageable.
- There is no major change—such as caring for a baby or an aging parent, or starting a new job—anticipated in

the next several weeks or already underway in your life.
- You are sufficiently dissatisfied with your health that you can make change a priority right now. You are holding this book because you want to cultivate more wellness, not because someone else thinks you should.

Be honest with yourself. If you don't feel ready, that's okay. Come back to this book when you are prepared to take action. Anything we undertake with halfhearted commitment will yield halfhearted results (and full-blown disappointment).

Change can be scary. We are biologically wired to avoid the unknown. Like Tonya, I have stood at the crossroads of desiring a change while, at the same time, feeling apprehensive about the repercussions of my dream coming true. I attribute my success to clear intentions, willingness to make sacrifices, playing to my strengths, and soliciting support from others to compensate for my kryptonite.

Whatever our journey, a little preparation can make all the difference in our experience. If you believe you're ready to take the first step, let's begin with a simple energy medicine technique.

The Focuser Technique

Once, a coworker who lived nearby convinced me that her route to work was better than mine. The next morning, I decided to try her way. My commute was so uncomfortable that, the following day, I resumed my old familiar route.

We should all feel grateful for the human survival instinct—(after all, you wouldn't be reading this book right now without it). But this invaluable aspect of our biology can interfere when we want to change established patterns of behavior. Our survival instinct prefers old familiar behaviors because the outcome is predictable. Been there. Done that. Still alive.

Engaging in a new behavior, however, jolts our survival instinct into full alert. It asks, "What is happening? Is this safe? Are you sure you want to do this?" If you have tried to make changes in the past only to find yourself reverting back to your old ways, now you know that you were battling primal human instinct.

What behaviors are automatic for you? Do you start and end every day the same way? Perhaps, like me, you follow the same route to work. Maybe you always reach for the same brand of paper towels in the grocery store or always order the same dish at your favorite restaurant. After all, you reason, I've gotten it before, and I know that I like it. How does it feel when you deviate from your established routine?

The Focuser Technique softens our natural reluctance to try something new. It also clears our mind of racing thoughts so we can think more clearly. Finally, this technique stimulates blood flow to the part of our brain where learning occurs. The Focuser will support you in your transformational journey to a healthier you. I recommend taking a few moments to practice The Focuser Technique every time you sit down to read this book and whenever you feel resistant to trying something new.

The steps are listed below—or you can follow along with me, using the video demonstration in the online companion.

1. Begin by sitting in a relaxed position with both feet flat on the floor. If it feels comfortable, close your eyes.
2. Rest the palm of one hand gently on your forehead. Use the other hand to cup the back of your head just above the neck. Imagine energy emanating from each palm, filling your skull with soft white light. Take five deep breaths in and out, through your nose.
3. Slowly reposition your hands until your fingertips are hovering over your eyelids and pointed toward your nose. Take a deep breath and slowly exhale.

4. Gently pull your hands outward until your fingertips are resting on your temples. Take a deep breath and slowly exhale.
5. From your temples, trace your fingertips around your ears and down your neck until your hands are resting on your shoulders with your fingertips on your back. Take another deep breath and slowly exhale.
6. Increase the pressure and drag your hands down to rest over your heart. Take another deep breath and slowly exhale.
7. Repeat Steps 3–6 two more times.

PART 2
MEET THE EIGHT INTENTIONS

THREE
THE DEMONSTRATED POWER OF INTENTION

BEGINNING IN 2007, investigative journalist and best-selling author Lynne McTaggart collaborated with Dr. Gary Schwartz and the University of Arizona's laboratory team to conduct a series of blind experiments on the power of intention.

In one study, they measured the impact of intention on seed germination and growth. Researchers in the lab divided 120 barley seeds into four groups of thirty seeds each. Volunteers in remote locations focused for ten minutes on the intention that their specific group of barley seeds would grow more rapidly over the next five days than the ninety seeds in three control groups. Following the intention session, researchers planted the seeds, not knowing which group of seeds the volunteers had sent intention to.

This experiment was repeated six times, including one instance with volunteers in Australia—850 miles away from the lab. Consistently, the intended-for seeds grew an average of a third of an inch more—a statistically significant result with a probability of coincidence at 0.7 percent.

In the ensuing decades, McTaggart has continued to partner with leading academic researchers to conduct dozens of experiments investigating the ability of mental intention to influence material reality. Her research substantiates the power of intention to heal damaged leaves, purify water, and reduce violence. Of the forty-one experiments completed to date, thirty-seven demonstrated statistically significant positive results.

Perhaps most impressive are the peace intention experiments McTaggart coordinated in Sri Lanka (2008), Afghanistan and Washington, D.C. (2012), and St. Louis, Missouri (2017). In the 2017 experiment, the intention was to reduce incidences of violent crime (rape, robbery, aggravated assault, and murder) in the Fairground neighborhood of St. Louis. Although overall crime increased 7 percent in the six months following the intention, violent crime fell by 43 percent.

More recently, McTaggart has been organizing people into small groups that send healing intention to a designated individual for ten minutes. In her book *The Power of 8*, published in 2017, McTaggart documents examples of miraculous healing—not only for the intended recipient, but also for the participants. I have experienced the power of intention firsthand as a member of a Power of 8 group. To learn more about McTaggart's work, including statistical analysis from the intention experiments, visit her website: LynneMactaggart.com.

Meet the Eight Intentions

We arrived in this lifetime with a promise in our virtual pocket: a life purpose that we aim to achieve while in this earthly form. Life is a treasure hunt to discover our intention and fulfill the promise.

As Mark Twain wisely informs us, "The two most important days in your life are the day you are born and the day you find out why." Some of us realize our purpose in childhood. Others arrive at the end of our days still searching.

There is a version of our life where our purpose is achieved. If we aren't moving toward it, we may have strayed off the path. Perhaps we allowed a misguided mindset to redirect our focus in the wrong direction. We may have plopped down along the wayside to nurse our wounds and neglected to resume our journey. Or, we may have become distracted by shiny objects that appeared to bring happiness but in reality weighed us down.

The eight intentions are a map to the path we are meant to be on. Bushwhacking our way out of the wilderness may not be easy, but the path is waiting for us if we do the work to find it. The eight intentions in this book are broad concepts, like guideposts for your life journey. Although I will give you specific examples of how to integrate them into your life, I encourage you to explore your own ways to apply them to your unique experiences.

1. I intend to cultivate resilience to stress.
2. I intend to elevate my vibrational frequency.
3. I intend to focus my attention on what is important.
4. I intend to embrace a growth mindset.
5. I intend to release energetic blockages.
6. I intend to nourish my body.
7. I intend to move my body every day.
8. I intend to connect with other people.

While I will introduce the intentions in sequence, each intention is one aspect of an integrated whole, like pieces of a jigsaw puzzle that fit together to create a picture. On any given day, we may have the opportunity to practice multiple intentions. For example, lowering our stress elevates our vibe, which enables us to focus on what is important, thereby improving our relationships. Or, moving our body improves our sleep, helping us to be more focused.

In my career as a project manager, every project began by documenting the desired goal or outcome. By industry definition, a project has specific criteria to achieve. Once that is accomplished, the project will conclude.

In some ways, the eight intentions resemble project goals;

they describe a desired future state. But unlike goals, these intentions are perpetual. There will be days when we fall short of our intentions. Perhaps stress overwhelms us, or we get caught up in emotions that lower our vibe. But every moment of every day is an opportunity to recommit to our intentions. Unlike a project, practicing the eight intentions never ends. After all, the Buddha did not stop meditating once he achieved enlightenment.

FOUR
INTENTIONAL RESILIENCE

I intend to cultivate resilience to stress.

ACCORDING to the American Psychological Association (APA), "Resilience is the process and outcome of successfully adapting to difficult or challenging life experiences, especially through mental, emotional, and behavioral flexibility and adjustment to external and internal demands."[1]

To me, the word "resilience" brings to mind a bop bag—an inflatable toy (often decorated with the image of a clown) that springs back to an upright position after being punched. New me is like a bop bag. Life still knocks me sideways sometimes, but because I have cultivated resilience to stress, I can quickly recover.

Intentional resilience involves mastering the skills that enable us to bounce back from the inevitable stresses of life. To learn how to cultivate resilience, let's begin by exploring how to recognize and manage the symptoms of stress.

Jaylen's Story

Jaylen lives in a scenic town nestled in the valley of a mountain range. The stream that meanders alongside the main street is peaceful except in springtime. That's when melting snow from the mountains above transforms the stream into a churning cauldron of muddy water, broken branches, and other debris. Jaylen still shudders when he recalls the year that a torrential rainstorm combined with the spring thaw forced the stream to spill over its banks. He was leaving for work one morning when he spotted a wall of water thundering down the street. Somehow, he made it back inside and up the stairs before the water surged through his front door. Now, every spring, Jaylen feels a sense of dread whenever rain is in the forecast. His heart beats faster and his stomach clenches as he considers what might have happened if he had not made it back to his house in time.

The Stress Response

Jaylen reacted quickly to the flash flood thanks to his stress response. The stress response is autonomic, meaning that we cannot consciously control it. Chemicals including adrenaline, cortisol, insulin, and cholesterol flood the bloodstream. Our heart rate accelerates while breathing becomes fast and shallow. As our body prepares for action—either to fight back or run away—all our available energy is redirected to muscles in the arms and legs. Basic functions such as cellular growth and repair, digestion, wound healing, and combating viruses cease to operate. Our field of vision narrows as we direct all our focus on the perceived threat. In his rush to escape, Jaylen did not need to notice that his grass needed mowing, for example. The part of our brain that helps us evaluate options and solve problems goes offline. Instead, the brain surrenders control to our reflex-oriented instinct, which reacts faster than the rational mind. Instinct enables us to hit the brakes when the driver in front of us swerves unexpectedly, yank our hand away from a hot stove, or dash to higher ground in the path of oncoming flood waters. Our body responds before our brain realizes what is happening.

Refer to the Symptoms of the Stress Response table to see how our physiological functioning changes when the stress response is triggered.

How much time do you spend in "Rest, Digest, and Heal" mode? Would you like to spend more time there?

What triggers the stress response for you? A lengthy to-do list and running late to an appointment are stressful for me. Take a moment to list your common stressors in your journal. We will come back to them later.

Nature designed the stress response for short-term use. As soon as we escape the threat, our body is supposed to revert to homeostasis or "rest, digest, and heal" mode. The physical activity of running away or fighting back clears the stress response chemicals from our bloodstream, allowing cellular growth, digestion, rational thinking, and immune system function to be fully restored. You may have seen nature shows where as soon as the antelope outruns the hungry lion, it resumes grazing peacefully as if nothing happened.

One of my clients has a small dog, Daisy, that barks at every little noise. Often it is hard to tell what sets her off; perhaps it's neighbors working in their yard, or the wind rustling the leaves in the trees outside the kitchen door. Because my client is elderly and lives alone, an alert dog like Daisy is a good safety measure —as long as she settles once her owner gives the all-clear signal. We want to train our stress response to behave like Daisy. It should switch into "fight or flight" mode when it senses danger and then stop barking and return to homeostasis once the situation is resolved.

Symptoms of the Stress Response

Homeostasis Rest, Digest, and Heal	Stress Response Fight or Flight
Primary chemicals in the blood include dopamine, oxytocin, and growth hormone. Blood chemistry is regulated as needed for sleep, digestion, and healing.	The blood is flooded with adrenaline, cortisol, cytokines, and pain-inhibiting chemicals. Glucose, insulin, and cholesterol are released to expedite energy supply to the muscles.
Heart rate, blood pressure, and respiration are at the body's typical resting rate.	Blood pressure and heart rate increase. Breathing becomes shallow and fast.
The body feels calm, safe, and open to emotions such as love and compassion.	The body is on high alert. The primary emotion is fear.
Eyes are relaxed and scanning the environment.	Pupils dilate. Our vision tunnels as our eyes lock on the perceived threat. The ability to hear certain frequencies may be impaired.
Energy is focused on digestion (absorption of nutrients), elimination of waste, cellular growth and repair, and immune system function.	Energy is redirected to the extremities (arms and legs) in preparation to fight or flee the threat. The immune and digestive systems are suppressed because the body does not want to expend energy combating infections/viruses or digesting food until the threat is resolved.
The brain uses experience, insight, and empathy in the prefrontal cortex (fore brain) for thinking and decision-making. The brain is open to receive new information (learning).	The brain relies on instinct and emotions in the limbic system (hind brain) because reflexes respond faster than executive functions.

The stress response is both a blessing and a curse. We tend to use the term "stress" to refer to distress, a form of stress that arises when we feel overwhelmed. But the stress response can also help us focus on a deadline, prepare for a presentation, or improve athletic performance. This beneficial form of stress, known as *eustress*, is often associated with personal growth.

We would not want to suppress our stress response even if we could. After all, the quick reaction triggered by Jaylen's distress response saved his life, while eustress motivates us to excellence in situations we find challenging yet rewarding.

Chronic Stress

One stressor can lead to another. For example, imagine that you oversleep one morning. When you finally wake up, your first surge of adrenaline launches you out of bed in a mad dash to get ready. In full-on fight-or-flight mode, you deviate from your typical morning routine, triggering additional releases of adrenaline every time you have to backtrack because you forgot something. As you rush to the car, you realize that the lunch you packed the night before is still on the kitchen counter, so you experience another stress influx as you run back inside to retrieve it. And when you finally arrive at work, you realize that your shoes don't match. Say hello to another dose of stress chemicals every time you suspect someone is looking at your feet.

Unfortunately, when it comes to most modern-day stressors, neither fighting nor fleeing are viable options. We can't physically wrestle an overflowing in-box or run away from mismatched shoes. As a result, residual stress chemicals are still circulating in our bloodstream when the next stressor hits. Think of a leaf kept aloft by an autumn wind. Every time it drifts down toward the ground, another gust tosses it high up into the air again. Like that leaf, chronic stress occurs when our body never fully transitions back to homeostasis before the stress response reactivates.

Over time, chronic stress—also known as anxiety—takes a toll on our mental, emotional, and physical well-being. With the nervous system constantly on alert, it is hard to concentrate and make informed decisions. Restful sleep is elusive. Joints and muscles ache from being tensed for action. Because the immune system is receiving fewer resources, we are more susceptible to catching viruses, and wounds take longer to heal. Digestion doesn't work smoothly, leading to gastrointestinal stress and cravings.

The symptoms of chronic stress are listed in the Chronic Anxiety Self-Assessment in the back of this book and the online companion. Take the assessment now, and then retake it again after each chapter. Use the Self-Assessment Tracker to compare your scores as you progress through the book.

False Alarm

Although the human body is constantly evolving, the stress response is still adjusting to modern society. Violence overseas, a vicious comment on social media, or slow-moving traffic can activate the stress response even though there is no threat to our physical safety.

Even our thoughts—recalling memories from the past (like an argument with your partner) or worries about the future (like paying your credit card bill on time)—can trigger the stress response. Our survival instinct reacts the same way to past memories, future worries, or an actual emergency unfolding in the present. That is why Jaylen's body experiences the symptoms of fight-or-flight when he hears that rain is in the forecast. His body is preparing for action even though he is in no immediate danger.

Refer to your list of common stressors. How many are false alarms; in other words, how many are not life-threatening? Although an overwhelming to-do list and showing up late to an appointment feel stressful for me, they aren't a matter of life and death.

Sara's Story

Sara was nine years old when the night terrors started. She was home from school due to contracting the COVID-19 virus from a classmate. It was early in the pandemic; there was still a lot of uncertainty regarding the severity of the virus. Both Sara and her parents were understandably worried, although her symptoms were mild.

As darkness descended and bedtime approached, Sara's worry escalated into despair. She irrationally feared that if she went to sleep, she might not wake up. Although her parents tried to reassure her, Sara was inconsolable, leading to a mostly sleepless night for everyone in the family. In the morning, Sara's mom called the pediatrician, who recommended that Sara "think positive thoughts." That seemed to help during daylight hours, but Sara's fear returned again as bedtime approached. As her parents soon discovered, a terrified child cannot will herself into optimism any more than stressed-out old me could will myself into calmness. After a second sleepless night, Sara's mom contacted me.

Sara's night terrors were the result of a stress response in overdrive. In Healing Touch, we have techniques to remove unwanted energy from our client's biofield much the way that a lint brush removes cat fur from my dressy black pants. My goal as an energy healer was twofold: First, restore Sara's system to homeostasis, and second, teach her how to manage her stress response going forward.

After setting up my table in their living room, I invited Sara to lie down. She chose to sit upright instead—an indication that she was too agitated to relax. In my initial assessment, I detected buzzy energy around her head. To clear Sara's mind of racing thoughts, I positioned my hands on either side of her head with the intention of sending white light energy between my palms—just as you learned in the Focuser Technique. As Sara relaxed, she laid down on the table and her chattiness quieted. Next, I opened the energy centers in the sole of each foot before raking stressful energy down the length of her body and out through her feet. Finally, I taught Sara to use the Intentional Breathing Technique to soothe herself when the anxiety returned.

After our first energy healing session, Sara slept through the night. After a few more sessions, Sara told me, "Thank you, but I can manage on my own now." She was right; that was over three years ago, and the night terrors have not returned.

Intentional Breathing

Intentional breathing is easy to master and can be practiced anywhere, anytime—whether driving a vehicle, sitting in a meeting at work, or lying sleepless in bed staring at the ceiling. As Sara demonstrated, it is so easy a child can do it.

As we learned earlier, one symptom of the stress response is rapid and shallow breathing as the body prepares to fight back or run away. Long, slow intentional breathing is perhaps the most powerful method to counteract the stress response, as it reassures the brain that it can stop ringing the alarm bells. Imagine your brain thinking, "Huh! If our breathing is relaxed, then everything must be okay now." Like my client's dog, Daisy, our system reverts to "rest, digest, and heal" mode.

Three aspects of intentional breathing include moving the diaphragm, holding the breath, and an exhale that is longer than the inhale. The diaphragm is a thin, dome-shaped muscle in the torso. Attached to the ribs in the front and the vertebrae in the back, it stretches across the abdominal cavity, separating the heart and lungs from the intestines. When we inhale, the diaphragm should bow downward massaging the digestive organs. When we exhale, the diaphragm rounds upward pressing against the lungs to help expel carbon dioxide. This is called diaphragmatic (or belly) breathing because when we inhale fully, the downward movement of the diaphragm causes the belly to distend slightly outward.

If you pay attention to how other people breathe, you will see that many people breathe so shallowly that their bellies do not expand when they inhale. But with a little practice you will not be one of those people! Follow the steps below or practice along with me using the video in the online companion.

1. Safety first. Sit or lie down in a comfortable position. If you are a shallow breather, the extra oxygen might make you feel a little lightheaded.
2. Lightly rest one hand over your navel and the other hand in the center of your chest near your heart.
3. Mentally counting to four, take a slow deep breath, inhaling through your nose, feeling your belly rise as your diaphragm expands.
4. When you can't breathe in any more air, pause for seven seconds with your lungs filled to capacity.
5. Mentally counting to eight, exhale through your nose as slowly as you can. Keep exhaling until your belly shrinks back toward your spine and your diaphragm rises pushing all the stale air out of your lungs.
6. Again. Slowly inhale as deeply as you can. Pause. Then exhale slowly. Continue to breathe intentionally until you feel calm. Very good!

In the beginning, it may be challenging to count your breaths. The online companion document includes a link to a guided breathing practice that may be helpful while you are learning.

Not only is Intentional Breathing an excellent technique to restore homeostasis after a stress response, but a regular daily practice of Intentional Breathing also builds resilience to stress. Over time, you can recover from stress more quickly. Best of all, you will find that annoyances are less upsetting because you aren't allowing stress response chemicals to accumulate in your system.

Urgency Addiction

Early in my career, I worked on a help desk. My days were a constant stream of technical problems. By the time I resolved the first issue of the day, there were already three more people waiting for me to fix their problems. I felt a tremendous sense of obligation to respond quickly so people could get back to work. I often deprived myself of lunch and bathroom breaks so I could help as many people as possible. Kicking into high gear, revving on all cylinders, solving one issue after another, felt deeply rewarding.

A rush of adrenaline can be exhilarating. Recall that I used to start my day with self-imposed stress because being steeped in urgency felt normal. Swirling in a cyclone of busyness helped me feel productive. But there's a distinction between urgent tasks and important tasks. By prioritizing urgent activities, I ignored important activities like spending time with family and friends. Instead of taking time to rejuvenate, I would immerse myself in tackling tight deadlines at work. Seething with impatience, I would finish people's sentences if they took too long to express themselves. I deceived myself into thinking that a steady infusion of stress hormones was beneficial, even though it was ruining my health.

Our bodies can become so accustomed to the rush of stress hormones that we seek out opportunities to experience it. People bungee jump off bridges, skydive out of airplanes, or crowd into theaters to watch horror movies.

Urgency addicts are always in search of a crisis to resolve. My old manager, Jill, regularly stirred up trouble at work. She would exaggerate a simple misunderstanding between two coworkers into a complicated drama involving everyone on the team. Then Jill would swoop in like a superhero, extinguishing the fire that she herself had ignited before running to tell her boss how she had saved the day. As annoying as her behavior was, I can understand why she did it. Jill would become bored with her day-to-day responsibilities. She craved excitement. Tackling an urgent issue gave Jill such a sense of satisfaction that she couldn't resist the urge to create a crisis to resolve.

If you think you might be addicted to urgency, here are some things to consider:

- Do you constantly rush from one thing to another?
- Do you have notifications turned on for email and social media posts?
- Are you constantly checking your phone?
- Do you equate checking a lot of items off your to-do list with having a meaningful day?
- Do you prioritize a crisis at work over spending time with family?
- Do you find it hard to spend a day relaxing?
- Do you often make mistakes in your rush to respond immediately?
- Do you rush through each task in your eagerness to tackle the next one?
- Do you feel bored when there's no crisis to solve?
- Do you exaggerate the urgency of an issue so you feel more satisfaction when you resolve it?

If you answered *yes* to many of the questions above, your body may have become addicted to the rush of adrenaline. Breaking the craving for urgency requires intentional introspection, but it can be done. For me, I eventually realized that my need to be productive and solve problems filled a hole in my self-esteem by giving me a sense of purpose. Spend time with your journal exploring the source of your urgency addiction.

Unfortunately, urgency addiction is not harmless. Spending too much time in stress response mode denies our body adequate time to rest, digest, and heal. As we try to balance expectations between home and work, we need to ask ourselves whether we are allowing self-imposed urgency to compound our stress level.

Our stress level affects the stress levels of people around us. Jill's urgency addiction affected not only her own health but also that of the colleagues unfortunate enough to be swept up in her theatrics. We can do the opposite and lower the stress levels of other people by radiating our own calmness, as well. As you build resilience by practicing intentional breathing, people in your vicinity will absorb your peacefulness.

The Gamut Point Technique

Do you know someone like Jill who radiates so much nervous energy that you feel stressed just being around them? Here's a subtle technique you can use whenever you sense your nervous system sliding into fight-or-flight mode. Follow the instructions below or check out the video in the online companion.

1. Begin by practicing a few rounds of practicing Intentional Breathing.
2. Locate the gamut point by placing the tip of your index finger between the base of the ring and pinky fingers. Then slide your index finger along the back of your hand until you detect the point where the bones of those two fingers meet in a "V" shape.
3. Press, rub, or tap the gamut point with your index finger using firm yet gentle pressure.
4. Continue holding the gamut point and breathing until calm spreads throughout your body.

Note: It doesn't matter which hand you hold. You can switch hands at any time. The beauty of this technique is that no one knows what you are doing.

Our Two Brains

An impressive brick mansion sits atop the summit of a gently rolling hill near the entrance to my neighborhood. A much smaller house used to grace the top of the hill. When the current owners bought it, they built their mansion around the tiny structure instead of tearing it down and building from scratch. The analogy of my neighbors' mansion is helpful for understanding the basic anatomy of the human brain.

Neuroscience is a complex topic, and our knowledge of the brain continues to evolve; researchers are still debating the divisions between various structures and functions. Instead of exploring anatomical terms that are still evolving, let's consider our brain as an old small house that someone built a mansion around.

The original portion of our brain sits at the top of the spinal column. Built for survival, this reflex-oriented brain mostly reacts without thinking. Sense a threat, move away. Sense a pleasure, move toward it. Sense food, eat it. It's the part of our brain that instinctively yanks our hand back from a hot stove without thinking. The doctor taps your knee with a rubber mallet and your leg jerks; hence the phrase "knee-jerk reaction."

As human skulls evolved, our expanding foreheads created space for our brains to develop physically and functionally. Neural connections in the newer section integrate with the primitive portion much as electrical wiring in my neighbors' mansion runs seamlessly through the original walls. The rational portion of our brain residing behind our forehead performs executive functions, giving us the ability to control impulses, evaluate options, and solve complex problems. It enables us to feel empathy for others and allows for metacognition (the ability to think about our thinking). Scientists estimate that the rational portion of our brain doesn't fully mature until sometime between the ages of twenty and thirty years old. So, there may be a biological reason when a teenager doesn't anticipate the consequences of their actions.

When we feel safe, our rational brain dominates. When the stress response is triggered, reflex mode takes the steering wheel as executive functioning slips into the passenger seat. The rational brain lacks the processing speed of the original model. From a survival perspective, we don't need to waste time rationalizing the pros and cons of running when we are in the path of oncoming flood waters. Our life depends on an immediate reaction.

Scammers try to trick us into reacting from our reflex brain. For example, we've all gotten one of those emails that appears to have been sent from Amazon indicating that our credit card is about to be charged $3,000. "Click the link below to cancel the order," it says. Since our reflex brain responds faster than our rational brain processes, the scammers are hoping we click the link before our rational brain questions the legitimacy of the email.

For the past several years, we have collectively experienced repeated stressors. First, there was uncertainty about how to protect ourselves from COVID-19. As pandemic fears eased, there were concerns about the economy. Shuttered factories meant supplies were not keeping pace with demand, leading to rising prices. Schools attempted to pivot to online learning, but the results were less than stellar. Isolated at home, we lost touch with our social support networks.

Even though the pandemic is in our rearview mirror, we have fresh stressors. Prices remain high. When classrooms reopened, the learning loss became apparent. Social groups we belonged to before the pandemic may not have resumed meeting. Across the globe, people are experiencing devastating losses from major storms, wildfires, droughts, and violence.

As these stressors mount, our survival-oriented reflex brain revs into overdrive. Many people report feeling worried, overwhelmed or angry most of the time. As a result, they are more likely to knee-jerk react than compassionately respond. To restore a sense of safety and predictability, they seek to control circumstances and other people.

Although differences of opinion are nothing new, people who are not part of "our tribe" seem more threatening when we don't feel safe. People have reacted with violence when a stranger drives up their driveway or knocks on their door. Despite the triggering news reports, most of us are not in any immediate danger—but our reflex brain doesn't know that.

How has your life changed since the pandemic? Is your default stress level higher than it used to be?

Cultivating resilience insulates us from the stress-inducing chaos around us. Practiced daily, techniques like the Focuser, Intentional Breathing, and the Gamut Point Technique free us from the confines of our reflex brain so our rational brain can respond calmly and thoughtfully to life's challenges. I encourage you to practice these techniques every day and teach them to others so we as a society can cultivate resilience to needless worries and fearmongering.

How to Cultivate Intentional Resilience

Intentional Resilience is the first intention because reducing your stress prepares you for the other seven intentions. We are better able to learn, practice, and apply new information when we feel safe, relaxed, and well-rested.

Here are some steps you can follow as you work to cultivate Intentional Resilience.

1. Write this chapter's intention (*I intend to cultivate resilience to stress*) on a piece of paper and tape it to your bathroom mirror. Take a moment every morning to decide how you will practice the intention in the

day ahead. At the end of the day, congratulate yourself for taking action to cultivate your personal power.
2. Pick a point in your existing daily routine to practice the Intentional Breathing technique for two minutes at least twice every day. Use the Technique Practice Tracker sheet in the back of the book to track your progress.
3. In addition to your daily practice, use the Intentional Breathing Technique to mitigate the stress response whenever it happens.
4. Make note of specific situations, interactions, or times of day when your stress is elevated. Use your journal to explore why that is and identify solutions to remedy the situation.
5. When stress interferes with your ability to concentrate, or you feel overwhelmed, use the Focuser Technique to clear your mind.
6. Consider whether you have an urgency addiction. If you do, use your journal to investigate the cause and identify solutions to remedy the situation.
7. Recognize the symptoms of stress in others. When people lash out, realize that they may be reacting from their original brain and respond compassionately.
8. As you become calmer, practice radiating calm energy to the people around you.
9. Use the Gamut Point Technique for quick stress relief in the moment.
10. Share these stress-relieving techniques with loved ones and friends.
11. Monitor your stress level by asking yourself throughout the day, "How would I rate my anxiety right now on a scale of one to five?"
12. Retake the Chronic Anxiety Self-Assessment. Log your score in the Self-Assessment Tracker to monitor changes in your stress level over time.

FIVE
INTENTIONAL VIBES

I intend to elevate my vibrational frequency.

WHAT DO we mean when we refer to "vibes?" When we say that a restaurant has a tropical vibe or a song has an uplifting vibe, we are referring to the atmosphere or the way that something makes us feel. Vibes can also refer to our intuition warning us to stay away from a dubious investment or encouraging us to take a leap of faith.

In the context of this intention, however, "vibes" refers to measurable electromagnetic waves of energy emanating from all living beings. The frequency of those vibrations—or vibes—affects not only how we feel, but also our overall health.

Intentional vibes involve tuning in to our energetic frequency and choosing behaviors, situations, and people that maximize our energetic potential.

We Are Vibrations

My five senses trick me into thinking that I am my physical body. My eyes are my windows to the world around me. I look down and see my hand, which lifts the shampoo bottle to my nose so I can inhale its floral scent. When I am driving, my ears alert me to an approaching fire truck before it is close enough to see.

But there is so much more than what we can see, hear, and touch. Quantum physics teaches that everything is energy vibrating incessantly in ascending and descending waves.

Despite what your five senses tell you, nothing—including your body and the chair you are sitting in—is solid and fixed. The chair is composed of atoms, which are a collection of subatomic particles held together by an electromagnetic charge. The atoms are 99.99999 percent energy.

Even your body is changing every second. Your next inhale will replace the air in your lungs right now. Your bloodstream is transporting nutrients to hungry cells while metabolic by-products are being trucked away for elimination.

While it is tempting to dismiss the existence of something we cannot sense, consider that gravity anchors us to a spinning planet whirling through space even though we cannot perceive the motion of Earth. The vibrations of our voice travel on invisible radio waves when we engage in a cell phone conversation with someone miles away.

What we interpret as solid objects are actually composed of atoms vibrating so slowly that they appear solid to us. But, when scientists break open the tiniest subatomic particles, they release the waves of energy tucked inside.

Referred to as *chi* in Tai Chi or *prana* in yoga, all living beings are animated by an intangible life force energy that scientists can measure six or more feet from the surface of our skin. In 1992, the National Institutes of Health (NIH) adopted the term *biofield* for this "massless field, not necessarily electromagnetic, that surrounds and permeates living bodies and affects the body."[1]

Imagine that you are surrounded by an invisible cocoon of energy. Ideally, our biofield is smooth and equidistant around the physical body—top to bottom, back to front, and side to side. In HT, we check for anomalies in the biofield before a session, and again afterward to confirm that our interventions have restored a balanced flow.

People's biofields can feel hot, dense, or sharp. In Sara's situation, her worry felt like a buzzy energy around her head. Following Tonya's hip replacement surgery, the sensation of a breeze moving across my palm indicated a tear in the biofield known in HT as an *energy leak*.

I have encountered biofields that are so elevated that the lower edge aligns with the client's knees—a foot or more above the ground. These people usually describe feeling caught up in swirling thoughts.

On a few occasions, someone's biofield was so off-center that it reminded me of the cliché "beside myself" that people use when they feel overwhelmed. Their biofield literally was beside their physical body. Sometimes, this may be the result of extreme impact—such as a fall or a vehicle accident.

You can feel your own biofield by holding your hands in front of you with palms facing each other. Slowly bring your hands toward and away from each other (without touching) several times and note how it feels when your palms come close. You may detect heat, pressure or resistance. Closing your eyes may help you tune into the sensation. How would you describe what you feel?

If you have a willing partner, experiment bringing your palms near theirs beginning from about eighteen inches away. Then, staying about six inches away, try moving your hands around their body. If they have a painful area like a headache or a cranky knee, see if the space around that area feels different to you. It may take a little practice, but I believe everyone can learn to feel biofields.

Some people see biofields with ease. I am still developing this skill but I *can* see the field around my hand when I hold it at arm's length against a white background in dim light. As I slowly move my hand while gazing at it with a relaxed focus, I can detect a halo, or aura, around it.

Flowing Rivers and Spinning Wheels

The energy in our biofield is constantly moving. Some of the energy circulates throughout our body in rivers called *meridians*. There are twelve primary meridians winding throughout the human body. Sometimes, a meridian splits into two or more branches. Sometimes, meridians will connect to other meridians. As these meridians loop through the body, they may intersect with a particular organ, which gives the meridian its name. The pathways of the primary meridians are described in the table.

The Primary Meridians

Meridian	Path
Heart	From the heart where it branches through the diaphragm to the small intestine, or up the throat to the lower eye, or across the chest to the armpit and down the inner arm to the tip of the little finger.
Lung	From just above the navel, through the large intestine, diaphragm, stomach, lungs, throat, shoulder, and arm, to the outer tip of the thumb.
Kidney	From the outside of the little toe, under the foot, along the arch to the inner ankle, through the heel, up inside of the leg to tailbone, up the spine to the kidney before branching to the bladder, up the chest to the collarbone or to the liver, diaphragm, lungs, and throat to the root of the tongue.
Liver	From the big toe, across the top of foot, up the inside of the leg, liver, and gallbladder before branching to the lung meridian, up the throat to the eyes, before branching across the cheek to the lips, or across the forehead to the crown of the head and connecting to the Governing meridian.
Governing	From the pelvis, up the spine, over the top of the head, and down the face to the upper lip.
Bladder	From the inner corner of the eye, up the forehead to the crown of the head before descending down the back of the neck, the buttocks, the back of the legs, and along the outer edge of the foot to the small toe.
Gallbladder	From the outer corner of the eye, to above the ear, down the side of the neck to the armpit, down and forward to the ribcage, down and back to the side of the waist, down to the front of the hip, down the outer side of the leg, and across the top of the foot to the tip of the fourth toe.

Meridian	Path
Spleen	From the big toe, up the inside of the leg, moving to the front of the leg above the knee, up the front side of the torso to a spot even with the shoulder, then down to the armpit.
Small Intestine	From the outer tip of the little finger, up the outer arm, across the back of the shoulder to the spine before branching to the heart, the diaphragm, the stomach, and the small intestine, or up the side of the neck, to the center of the cheek ending in front of the ear.
Large Intestine	From the tip of the index finger, up the outer edge of the arm, across the shoulder blades to the spine, before branching either to the lungs, the diaphragm, and the large intestine, or up to the neck, across the face to the side of the nose.
Stomach	From below the eye, past the outer corner of the mouth to the center of the jaw before branching either to the side of the forehead or down the front of the torso and the leg to the tip of the second toe.
Triple Warmer	From the tip of the ring finger, up past the back of the elbow to the back of the shoulder, around to the front side of the neck, up behind and over the ear to in front of the ear before ending at the temple.

In addition to the rivers of energy, our biofield contains spinning vortices of energy called *chakras*, which is the Sanskrit word for "wheel." The chakras resemble tornadoes, with the base originating in the physical body and widening outward away from it. The number of chakras varies by school of thought. For example, the ancient Hindu system of medicine— Ayurveda—identifies seven primary chakras.

In HT, we evaluate the movement of the client's seven primary chakras, as well as smaller chakras in the arms and legs, before and after a session. An open chakra spins smoothly in a clockwise circle. A chakra that wobbles in an elliptical direction or is motionless requires interventions to restore a balanced spin.

The table provides a high-level introduction to how the primary chakras affect our wellbeing.

The Primary Chakras

Chakra	Description
Root	Associated with the color red and the element of earth, the root chakra originates at the base of the spine funneling like an inverted tornado pointed downward toward our feet. It is related to our survival, our sense of purpose, belonging, and the will to live. A healthy root chakra helps us feel grounded and stable.
Sacral	Associated with the color orange and the element of water, the sacral chakra originates a few inches below the navel. It is associated with sensuality, desire, and procreation. A healthy sacral chakra enables us to move with ease and enjoy pleasure without guilt. *Like all the chakras (except the root and the crown), the sacral chakra extends in front of and behind our body like two tornadoes joined at the base.*
Solar Plexus	The color is yellow, and the element is fire. The solar plexus originates a few inches above the navel. A healthy solar plexus supports our autonomy as individuals, our self-esteem, self-discipline, and personal power.
Heart	Associated with the color green and the element of air, the heart chakra is near the sternum bone at the level of our physical heart. A healthy heart chakra enables us to love ourselves and others, feel empathy, and express compassion.

Chakra	Description
Throat	Colored bright blue with the element of sound, the throat chakra resides at the base of our neck. Communication is the theme—whether expressing ourselves or listening to others. A healthy throat chakra enables us to find our voice and express our creativity.
Brow	Associated with indigo and the element of light, the brow chakra originates between, and slightly above, our eyebrows. It supports our perception, imagination, intuition, and spiritual insight. A healthy brow chakra opens our mind to learning, clarity, and wisdom.
Crown	Colored violet, the crown chakra is associated with the element of thought. It originates at the top of—or slightly above—the skull and funnels upward toward the heavens. A healthy crown chakra supports our ability to be open-minded and visionary. It connects us to our higher power.

Interestingly, there appears to be anatomical evidence for both the meridian system and the chakras. Using tracer dyes, computed tomography (CT) scans, and dissection, researchers discovered a thread-like system of vessels that loop through the fascia (connective tissue) intersecting with various organs. These vessels follow the routes of the meridians as documented by practitioners of Traditional Chinese Medicine (TCM) thousands of years ago. Scientists named this system the primo-vascular system (PVS) in 2010.[2] In addition to other healthful substances, primo-vessels carry electrical signals and life-sustaining multipotent stem cells.

Six of the primary chakras are located near "junction boxes" of intersecting nerves known as *neurological plexuses*. Located in the center of the brain, the choroid plexus is near the origin point of the Brow chakra. The Throat chakra is near the cervical and brachial plexuses. The Heart chakra is near the cardiac plexus. The celiac plexus, also known as the solar plexus, is located near the Solar Plexus chakra. Finally, the superior hypogastric plexus is near the Sacral chakra, while the Root chakra is in the vicinity of inferior hypogastric plexus. Missing from the list is the Crown chakra, which—according to some schools—originates outside the physical body above the apex of our skull. The fact that nerves carry electrical signals may explain why the biofield energy is more discernible in the vicinity of the plexuses.

Imagine the fast-moving water in the middle of a river. The water is churning, energized, constantly rejuvenated. A leaf that drifts down into the river is swiftly carried away by the current. If a storm topples a tree into the river, the flow of water is obstructed. The water moves slowly; in some places, it barely moves at all. If a leaf settles here, it will rot in the still water. The quiet pools along the decaying tree trunk become stagnant, dank, and oxygen-deprived. There's a foul stench.

The energy in our biofield should flow freely like an unimpeded river. But just as the fallen tree disrupts the river's current, low-frequency vibes create congestion in our biofield. Low vibes can be the result of physical injury, psychological trauma, chronic anxiety, or even emotions like hate, regret, and blame. Eventually, the reduction of life-force energy in the affected area manifests as physical symptoms.

Let's say I am feeling uncertain about a pending life change. According to *You Can Heal Your Body* by Louise Hay, my trepidation interferes with the flow of energy in my legs—the part of our body that moves us forward.[3] Over time, I begin to experience pain in my knees, which leads to joint damage, then physical therapy, and perhaps surgery. But, if I acknowledge my uncertainty and remind myself that I have successfully navigated major changes in the past, the energy flow is restored before damage occurs.

Refer back to your list of chronic stressors. How does it feel when you experience the stress response? Where do you feel it in your body? Stressed-out old me always felt tightness in my shoulders and bowel.

What chakra is closest to where you feel stress? What aspect of our well-being is governed by that chakra? Is it associated with the situation that is causing your stress?

How does that area of your body feel when you are in "rest, digest, and heal" mode? Does the stress sensation disappear entirely?

Bring to mind something that makes you angry. Anger is a low-vibe emotion. Where do you feel it in your body?

Now think of someone you love. Love is a high-vibe emotion. Where do you feel love in your body?

Just like everything else, our thoughts and emotions are also vibrating energy. No doubt you've experienced knowing what someone is thinking or feeling without them uttering a word. Not only are the electromagnetic signals of the heart and brain detected by every cell in our body, but they are also broadcast to people around us.

Our heart is sending the most powerful signals. Using electrocardiogram (ECG) and electroencephalogram (EEG) devices, scientists have discovered that the amplitude of the heart's electrical field is about sixty times greater than the brain's. Using a magnetocardiogram (MCC), scientists discovered that the heart's magnetic field is 100 times stronger than the brain's and has been measured up to six feet away from our physical body in all directions.

Researchers have developed technology that can identify a subject's emotions by analyzing heart rhythm data collected via ECG. In 2016, scientists at MIT developed a wireless version—nicknamed EQ-Radio. A review conducted in 2023 identified over ten different emotion detector devices in development that can identify the vibes of surprise, sadness, anxiety, passion, joy, shame, hope, fear, disgust, anger, gratitude, intimacy, trust, pain, confidence, and relaxation.

This technology demonstrates that our emotions radiate

outward for others to receive and interpret. The reason we cannot do it all the time is that we have to be tuned to the other person's frequency, just as we must tune a radio to the desired frequency to listen to the station that we want. The next time you interact with someone, try tuning into their vibes. Notice how the vibes you detect align with the words that they are saying.

Linda's Story

When Linda checked in for her surgery on Monday, the doctor predicted that she would spend one night in the hospital and go home the following day. But one night stretched into two, and then three, as the doctors struggled to ease Linda's postoperative pain. When I entered her hospital room on Wednesday evening, Linda was propped up in her bed, furrows of misery etching deep creases into her pale face.

As I extended my hands toward her, I noticed the space around Linda felt dense and heavy. When I moved my hands in the direction of her incisions, my palms detected heat and a jagged sharpness—like broken glass. Holding my hands about two feet away from Linda, I began to slowly and gently move my outstretched fingers along the length of her body, from above her head to below her feet. Although my hands appeared to be moving through empty air, it felt as if I was pulling my fingers through a thick mat of tangled hair. Over the course of thirty minutes, the resistance slowly gave way.

By this time, Linda had fallen into a deep sleep, which is a sign that self-healing has begun. Color returned to her face as the creases softened, but there was still more work for me to do. I held my motionless hands about twelve inches away from her incisions. I felt the energy of pain draining out of Linda's body and across my palms like water streaming from an open faucet.

The nurse came in, so I lowered my arms and stepped out of her way. When she saw Linda sleeping peacefully, the nurse came to an abrupt halt. "I don't know what you are doing," she said to me, "but keep doing it. She hasn't looked like that since she got here. I'm going to hold off on administering her next dose of pain medication." When the flowing sensation stopped, I repositioned my hands slightly, inviting fresh energy to flow from the space around us into Linda's body. Then I smoothed my hands around the area of the incisions to repair the hole in her biofield. In closing, I set the intention for her continued healing. Linda went home the next day.

Biofield Therapy

Although Linda's surgery may have saved her life, the surgeon's actions—cutting her body open and removing tissues—was as disruptive to her energy flows as a concrete dam. The stitches and swelling were evidence of the physical damage from surgery. What was not visually apparent was the gaping wound in Linda's biofield allowing tiny bits of her life-force energy to trickle out. Residual anesthesia was dampening her energy flow even further. The biofield damage interfered with her body's ability to initiate the healing process. By administering HT interventions, I was able to repair her biofield. With the flow of energy restored, Linda fell into a deep sleep as her body began the process of healing.

Biofield therapy—also known as energy medicine—refers to various healing modalities designed to restore unimpeded flow of energy in our biofield, thereby maximizing our overall well-being. Examples of biofield therapies include HT, Therapeutic Touch, reiki, acupuncture, and qigong.

Biofield therapies have been practiced for thousands of years. Once considered woo-woo, acupuncture is now recommended by the NIH to treat several types of pain as well as irritable bowel syndrome, seasonal allergies, fibromyalgia, incontinence, and nausea associated with surgery or chemotherapy. Some insurance companies even pay for acupuncture treatments. According to my acupuncturist, leaving a hair-thin needle inserted into an acupuncture point for about twenty minutes restores the energetic flow in the meridian.

In HT, we use the energetic vibrations emanating from our hands to move our client's energy—clearing away congestion, reenergizing flows, and sealing leaks. Developed in the 1980s by a Navy nurse, Janet Mentgen, the Healing Touch Program is endorsed by the American Holistic Nurses Association, the Canadian Holistic Nurses Association, and the Watson Caring Science Institute. Healing Touch is taught in nursing schools and offered to patients in hospitals, Veterans Administration (VA) facilities, and outpatient cancer treatment centers. On my website are videos produced by medical facilities that have added HT to their patient care protocols. As one of the nurses says in the VA's video, the best way to understand HT is to experience a session firsthand.

HT for Animals (HTA), which modifies HT interventions for use with animals, was introduced in 1996. In HTA, we clear an animal's biofield with sound waves from tuning forks in addition to using our hands.

Conventional Western medicine is developing devices that work on the same principle of healing through vibrations. In 1979, the FDA approved the clinical use of Pulsed Electromagnetic Field (PEMF) devices, which generate spurts of magnetic waves to stimulate bone growth in fractures that do not respond to standard treatment. According to a 2003 article in the journal *Techniques in Orthopaedics*, the magnitude and quality of energy emitted from the hands of Therapeutic Touch practitioners was comparable to the waveforms from a PEMF device.[4]

The Safe and Sound Protocol (SSP) uses sound waves to treat symptoms of depression, learning difficulties, sleep issues, and more by calming the fight-or-flight response. Sonu is an FDA-approved wearable device that uses sound waves to break up nasal congestion. Histotripsy uses soundwaves to eradicate cancer. In 2023, the FDA approved histotripsy for the treatment of inoperable liver tumors, but other forms of cancer may be added in the future.

Similar to traditional medicine, biofield therapies offer our body a boost when it is too depleted to heal on its own. For the best possible outcome, biofield therapies should be used in conjunction with conventional medicine, as they are complementary—not alternative—approaches.

Where's the Evidence?

Anyone who has not experienced energy medicine firsthand may be skeptical. "Where's the scientific evidence?" they ask.

Lack of funding is a key impediment to any form of scientific analysis. It's expensive to conduct medical research, particularly the gold standard—randomized controlled trials (RCTs). Funding is more available for a marketable product, such as a drug or a medical device, that will yield a return on investment. Primary sources of medical research funding, such as pharmaceutical companies, are disincentivized to study biofield therapies because the economics of health care could shift dramatically if demand for their products declined. Additionally, required aspects of RCTs—such as precisely measured dosages—don't apply to biofield therapies.

Recognizing the need for consistency in biofield therapy research, "Guidelines for Reporting Clinical Trials" was published in the peer-reviewed journal *Global Advances in Integrative Medicine and Health* in 2024.[5] Recommendations include documenting factors such as the healer's years of experience, the distance between the healer's hands and the client, the techniques used, length of the session, and whether the session was conducted in person or remotely. These standards will facilitate cross-study analysis and replication of biofield therapy research going forward.

That said, the Consciousness and Healing Initiative maintains a database of over 400 biofield therapy research papers on their website. Included in the database:

- A pilot study with over 100 dialysis patients found that HT reduced fatigue by 46 percent, pain by 68 percent, stress and anxiety by 49 percent, and depression by 84 percent. (2017) [6]
- An RCT involving 123 active-duty military, concluded that HT, along with guided imagery, was more effective in relieving symptoms of post-traumatic stress disorder (PTSD) than standard treatments (cognitive behavioral therapy, biofeedback, relaxation training, and—in many cases—medications). (2012)[7]
- A clinical trial of 237 patients undergoing cardiac bypass surgery found that HT reduced anxiety and the length of hospital stay. (2008)[8]

Skeptics question whether biofield therapies work due to the placebo effect; in other words, people feel better because they *expect* to feel better. While this may be a valid concern for human studies, it does not explain why animals respond positively to interventions used in Healing Touch for Animals.

Paul's Story

Paul had recently received a knee replacement. In assessing his biofield after surgery, I could not detect any life-force energy in Paul's new left knee. That part of his leg felt energetically disconnected from the rest of his leg—like a dead zone between cell-phone towers. It was as if by removing the knee joint, a section of the energy river connecting Paul's femur to his tibia had been scooped out.

Resting one hand above and the other hand below Paul's artificial knee, I intended for the energy to connect between my palms. After several minutes, the energy in Paul's leg started flowing again. At his follow-up appointment, the doctor indicated that Paul's healing was progressing faster than expected.

Although the energy flow in Linda's and Paul's biofields may have resumed on its own eventually, I believe that early restoration via HT interventions accelerated the self-healing process.

What is Grounding?

When our biofield is centered, the base extends about twelve inches below our feet to what some call the Earth star chakra. This connection allows the Earth's energy to flow upward through our feet, recharging us when we feel drained. We can also release excess energy into the Earth, just as your home's grounding wire discharges electrical system overloads.

In working with Sara and Linda, I raked excess energy—worry and pain—down the length of their body so it could drain out of their biofield through their feet. If someone is caught up in swirling thoughts, holding their feet can bring them back down to Earth.

Ancient humans lived in close contact with the ground—walking barefoot and sleeping on mats. In modern times, however, we rarely touch the earth directly. We live in buildings with cement foundations and walk on concrete sidewalks. When we venture out into nature, our feet are insulated by rubber-soled shoes. This separation weakens our connection with the Earth, making it harder to regulate our energy.

Recall how good it feels to take a barefoot stroll on the beach, dig in the garden or lie on a blanket in the grass. There's a scientific explanation. Just like us, this planet we call home radiates electromagnetic energy. Think of the electrical charge in lightning and the magnetic pull that makes a compass point northward. When we experience uninsulated contact with the surface of the Earth, the ground's charge neutralizes unstable atoms in our body that can lead to health problems such as cancer, autoimmune disorders, aging, rheumatoid arthritis, and cardiovascular and neurodegenerative diseases.

There are devices that connect to the grounding wire of your home's electrical system. Sitting or lying on these grounding mats allows your body to exchange energy with the Earth. My self-care includes sleeping on a grounding mat every night.

In HT training, we learn how to ground ourselves using intention. During a session, a client's energy will intermingle with my biofield. Ensuring that I am grounded before a session enables me to flush excess energy back into the earth. If I fail to properly ground myself first (which happened a lot when I was learning!), disruptions in a client's biofield can make me nauseous.

The Intentional Grounding Technique

Intentionally grounding yourself will take several minutes when you are first learning how to do it. With practice, though, you will be able to ground yourself in just a few seconds. The steps are listed below, or you can follow along with me using the video in the online companion.

1. Begin by sitting in a comfortable position with both feet flat on the floor.
2. Spend a few moments practicing Intentional Breathing.
3. Bring your awareness to the soles of your feet resting on the floor. There is an energy center—or chakra—on the bottom of each foot, a few inches below the second toe at the base of the ball of your foot. Rest your attention there while you continue to breathe with intention.
4. Imagine roots extending from the bottoms of your feet, through the foundation of the building you are in, deep into the earth. Picture your roots pushing

through soil, past stones and underground streams, and deep into the molten core of the planet. You might feel a slight tug as your body anchors to the earth.
5. There is a column of energy that runs vertically through the core of our body, called the *Hara*, or the line of intention. As you take a slow, deep inhalation through your nose, imagine revitalizing energy flowing up your roots, along the Hara, through the Crown chakra and up to the cosmos.
6. Exhale through your nose as slowly as you can while imagining swirling thoughts, negative emotions, and physical discomfort draining down the Hara and returning to the Earth through your roots.
7. Sit for a while, continuing to transfer energy to and from the earth, until you feel settled.

My Angry Shoulder

Energy vibrates in ascending and descending waves. The number of waves per second determines the frequency, which is measured in hertz (Hz). In his book *Power Versus Force,* Dr. David Hawkins introduces his Map of Consciousness. This map lists the frequency of emotions, from shame at 20 Hz to enlightenment at over 700 Hz. High-vibe emotions feel good; low-vibe emotions—not so much.

Vibrating at 150 Hz, anger is a low-vibe emotion. My anxiety was at its height in my forties. I was working full-time, going to school at night, raising two children, and volunteering as a troop leader. My husband's aging mother lived with us during this time. It felt to me that she was always voicing criticisms about my parenting, my cooking—even the clothes I wore. When the family went out together, she insisted that I sit in the backseat while she sat up front next to my husband. Once she gifted me a too-small skirt for my birthday explaining that it would be the motivation I needed to lose weight and reclaim my pre-motherhood figure. When I attempted to assert myself, she would cry and tell my husband that I was being mean to her. So, I resolved to remain silent, bottling up any words that might provoke another outburst.

After a time, I developed a painful stiffness in my right shoulder. Getting dressed or buckling the seat belt in my car was agony. The pain kept me awake at night. After a cortisone injection failed to elicit any relief, the doctor diagnosed me with a frozen shoulder. Months of painful physical therapy followed. About two years later, my left shoulder froze up, leading to another round with the same physical therapist. I asked her why this kept happening, but she didn't have an answer except to say that women are more susceptible to it.

When I began to study energy medicine years later, I finally understood. The shoulder is close to the throat chakra, the energy center that's related to finding our voice and speaking up for ourselves. Knowing what I know now, I believe that choking back my anger caused energetic congestion in my shoulders. In the twenty years since my mother-in-law passed, my shoulders have remained strong and healthy.

One tactic to protect yourself in a similar situation would be to have a heartfelt conversation with the other person. Use the energy medicine techniques you have learned to relax and ground yourself first so you can engage calmly.

In hindsight, I suspect that my mother-in-law's criticisms were well-intentioned. She was trying to mold me into the wife and mother she believed her son and grandchildren deserved. As we will discuss in a future chapter, I doubt that anything I could have said would have changed her opinion about my perceived shortcomings.

If I were to find myself in this situation again, I would use the Energetic Shield Technique to protect myself, in addition to Intentional Grounding to help me drain my frustration instead of stuffing it into my shoulders.

The Energetic Shield Technique

Just as it sounds like it would do, this technique forms a shield of protective energy around us so we can avoid taking on unhealthy energy from others. It may take several minutes to raise your energetic shield when you are first learning this technique, so use it in advance whenever you anticipate being in a vulnerable situation. The accompanying online companion includes a six-minute guided imagery meditation based on this technique.

Additionally, if you unexpectedly find yourself in a situation requiring immediate shielding, you can place one or both hands over your solar plexus chakra (just above your navel).

1. Stand or sit comfortably in a chair with both feet flat on the floor.
2. Spend a few moments practicing Intentional Breathing.
3. Imagine a field of energy surrounding you in all directions—your biofield. If you feel comfortable doing so, closing your eyes may help you tap into the sensation.
4. Focus your attention on the Crown chakra at the top of your head.
5. Imagine a stream of protective white light flowing into your Crown chakra, completely filling your biofield and wrapping you in a cocoon of safety.
6. Picture the outer edges of your biofield solidifying like a hard shell that nothing unwanted can penetrate.
7. Set the intention for ongoing defense by saying aloud or to yourself, "I intend to stay safe within my shield of protective energy."
8. When you feel ready, open your eyes and reconnect with the present.

Bill's Story

Bill went to his primary care physician complaining of pain in the upper left side of his chest. The doctor looked at Bill—a white man in his fifties—and suspected coronary heart disease. A stress test and blood work were ordered, but the doctor was perplexed when all the tests came back clear. With no angioplasty or bypass to be performed, there was nothing more for the doctor to do.

In Western medicine, doctors specialize in either physical or mental health. Yet, from an energy medicine perspective, segregating wellness into categories is like staring at Mona Lisa's hands while ignoring her smile. If the physician had delved into Bill's emotional state, he would have discovered that Bill's mother had recently passed. Bill was grieving. Whether from the death of a loved one or the end of a romantic relationship, grief hurts.

As the poet Robert Frost advises, "The best way out is always through." When it comes to emotions like grief, there is no way to avoid our feelings. As Bill allowed himself to experience his emotions, his grief eased, and so did his chest pain. Twenty years later, he has no recurring symptoms associated with coronary heart disease. If Bill had suppressed his grief—like I suppressed my anger with my mother-in-law—eventually, he might have developed a discernible heart issue.

Low-Vibes Are Inevitable

When I first encountered Hawkins' Map of Consciousness, I made the mistake of assuming that one should seek to dodge low-vibe emotions in the pursuit of high-vibration feelings. But as I delved deeper into his work, I realized that, although low-vibe emotions don't feel good, they are essential threads in the tapestry of life.

While it may feel unpleasant, the time we spend in the

troughs of low emotional vibes has value. First, a steady stream of rainbows and unicorns would be boring. The deliciousness of high vibes arises from the contrast to low vibes, just as the sunshine seems brighter after a cloudy week of rain. Second, just as diamonds are formed under pressure, adversity helps us grow. Finally, as in Bill's situation, grief is an inevitable part of a life filled with loving relationships. Allowing ourselves to fully experience low-vibe emotions is essential to moving past them. According to Hawkins, an episode of grief will run its course in about twenty minutes if we surrender to it.

Some of us have been conditioned to deny or repress emotions that don't feel good. Instead, honor the legitimacy of your emotions. We will explore this topic more deeply in the chapter on Intentional Release. Until then, use practices like Intentional Grounding—or, even better, uninsulated contact with the Earth—to balance your vibes.

Protecting Your Vibes

Friends and I were enjoying dinner out one night when conversation turned to a new TV show that everyone (except me) was watching. "Have you seen the latest episode?" someone asked. "Not yet!" someone else squealed. "Don't tell me what happens!" Their enthusiasm was contagious, so the following night I streamed the first episode. Brimming with violence, torture, deception, and addiction, the show was too dark for my taste. I made an intentional decision not to watch it for the sake of protecting my vibes.

Considering the incessant bombardment of low-vibe energy in nasty social media posts and dire predictions about the future of humanity, it is more important than ever to be choosy about the vibrational quality of the entertainment we consume.

No doubt you have experienced music that elevated your mood or a movie that tugged the heartstrings so forcefully the theater resounded with sniffling. While an occasional good cry provides an emotional release that leaves us feeling as cleansed as city streets after a rainstorm, a steady consumption of low-vibe entertainment is as unhealthy as a diet of ice cream and soda.

Because our brain does not distinguish between thinking about a dangerous situation and experiencing a real-life emergency, a violent scene in a movie triggers the stress response. As we discussed earlier, we can become addicted to the rush of stress hormones. Savvy producers tap into that adrenaline rush to attract audiences. But when we understand the health consequences associated with frequently ringing the alarm bells of fight-or-flight, we understand the importance of not exposing ourselves to unnecessary stress.

Think about the shows you watch, the games you play, and the music you listen to. Does it make you feel stressed or relaxed? Does it prompt you to smile or frown? Do the characters support or harm each other? Does it raise or lower your vibes?

How to Elevate Your Vibes

In the last chapter, we learned that cultivating resilience means learning to bounce back from—not eliminate—the stress response. Similarly, the purpose of Intentional Vibes is not to avoid low-vibe emotions. Instead, we want to tune into our vibes, unpack them, and process our emotions appropriately, freeing ourselves to return to the higher end of the frequency scale. Here are some tips for elevating your vibes:

1. Write this chapter's intention (*I intend to elevate my vibrational frequency*) on a piece of paper and tape it to your bathroom mirror. Take a moment every morning to decide how you will practice the intention in the

day ahead. At the end of the day, congratulate yourself for taking action to cultivate your personal power.
2. Spend time sensing the vibratory nature of your body and your environment by reminding yourself that nothing—even seemingly solid objects—is rigid or permanent.
3. Practice feeling your own biofield and the fields of other people.
4. As you move through each day, tune into your biofield and make note of how it feels. Is it flowing like an unimpeded river or are there areas that feel congested —even painful?
5. Monitor your vibrational frequency throughout the day by asking yourself, "How would I rate the frequency of my vibes right now? Do I feel serene, forgiving, scornful, or anxious? Why am I feeling this way?"
6. Pick a point in your existing daily routine to practice the Intentional Grounding Technique for at least two minutes every day. Use the Technique Practice Tracker in the back of the book to record your progress until it becomes a habit.
7. Practice the Intentional Grounding Technique whenever you feel depleted or overwhelmed.
8. When possible, spend time in uninsulated contact with the Earth. Go for a barefoot stroll, dig in the garden or sit on a blanket in the grass.
9. Choose entertainment (books, music, movies, etc.) that elevate your vibe.
10. When you experience pain or discomfort, note which chakra is in closest physical proximity of the feeling. Use your journal to explore whether you are experiencing any emotional or psychological challenges associated with the theme of that chakra.

11. If you want to learn more about the chakras, I recommend the works of Anodea Judith.
12. If you want to learn more about the benefits of grounding, I recommend the documentaries *The Earthing Movie* and *The Grounded,* both available free online.
13. You may find it helpful to reference Dr. Hawkins' Map of Consciousness, which is available in his books and online. I recommend his book *Letting Go: The Pathway to Surrender*.
14. Retake the Chronic Anxiety Self-Assessment. Log your score in the Self-Assessment Tracker to monitor changes in your stress level over time.

SIX
INTENTIONAL FOCUS

I intend to focus my attention on what is important.

IMAGINE that you are home one night when the power goes out. Fortunately, you have a flashlight within easy reach. As you move through your home, your attention is drawn to whatever objects appear in the beam of light. Everything else disappears in the darkness.

Our attention is like the flashlight beam—focusing on one thing and then another. Right now, your attention is on this page. In a moment, it could swing toward the roar of an airplane overhead, or a tickling sensation on the tip of your nose, and then back to the page. While it seems that you are simultaneously aware of this page, the airplane, and your itchy nose, this is an illusion created by your brain. In reality, we can focus only on one thing at a time, though our attention may be constantly shifting.

Intentional focus involves choosing where we direct our mental flashlight, with the understanding that what we choose to pay attention to affects both our stress level and the frequency of our vibes.

The Important Stuff

Chronically stressed, old perfectionist me tended to focus my mental flashlight on the gaps between how things were and how I thought they should be. I directed my attention toward my unkempt house, my excess weight, and urgent assignments at work. Focusing on the gaps distracted me from the important stuff in my life. Plus, when I said to myself, "I need to lose weight," I was lowering my vibe. Pause for a moment to consider what is important in your life. Where should you be pointing your flashlight?

Calm, new me has a succinct list:

- My physical, mental, spiritual, and energetic health.
- My purpose, which is to spread healing.
- My relationships with family and friends.
- My creative expression.

Although it is a short list, it encompasses the aspects of my life where I direct most of my attention. It's okay to have a long list initially, but over time, try to whittle it down to the essentials of what is most important to you. A long list would require a lot of erratic flashlight waving.

Grab your journal and create your own list. Phrase the items on your list from the perspective that raises your vibe; for example, if finances are important to you because resources are limited in your current situation, you might write down "my abundance" instead of "my debt." Then direct your focus to the prosperous aspects of your life apart from money.

Picture yourself pointing your flashlight of focus at each item on the list. Only include items that make you feel good when you focus on them.

Over the next week, notice where you are actually pointing your flashlight. Is it pointing in the direction of what is important, or are you paying too much attention to things that aren't on your list? If needed, write down some strategies for ensuring that your flashlight beam is shining in the right direction. More pointers are coming up later in this chapter!

The Pretzel Technique

When I was a child, my dad used to get so upset with me for breaking his rules that he would threaten to hit me "upside the head with a two-by-four" (he never actually did). Looking back, though, I wasn't trying to break the rules. Like most children, I wanted to please my parents and win their approval, but I literally lacked the mental capacity to always behave in accordance with their expectations. My flashlight of focus would point in the direction of something intriguing to my child brain, and Dad's rules were forgotten in the shadows beyond the beam.

If you are living in a state of chronic anxiety, you may struggle to stay focused on any one thing for very long. Like me when I was young, your mental flashlight may bounce around so wildly that you wonder whether intentional focus is accessible to you. Practicing the Focuser Technique that we learned at the beginning of this book helps calm racing thoughts so our brain can maintain focus.

Now let's learn another energy medicine technique that also disrupts the stress response and helps us to focus. The Pretzel Technique, or Balance Hook-up Technique, has the added benefit of balancing the flow of energy between the right and left hemispheres of the brain, helping us to feel grounded and centered.

This technique is also effective at helping rowdy children settle down. If there are children in your life, teach them how to "pretzel." Follow the instructions below or check out the video in the online companion.

1. Begin by sitting comfortably in a chair with both feet flat on the floor.
2. Cross your left ankle over your right ankle.
3. Reach both arms straight out in front of you parallel to the floor.
4. Rotate your arms so that the backs of your hands are facing toward each other and your thumbs are pointing toward the floor.
5. Cross the right arm over the left arm and interlace the fingers of both hands.
6. Pull your hands down and toward your body, and then back up so that your hands can rest near your collarbone.
7. (Optional) If you like, you may rest your chin on your thumbs.
8. In this position, practice Intentional Breathing for at least two minutes.

Note: If crisscrossing your arms is uncomfortable, an alternative is to cross your arms over your chest so that each hand rests below the opposite shoulder. This simple variation is good for children.

How Stress Affects our Focus

My friend Janet and I meet once a month to catch up over lunch. While Janet and I chat, my five sense organs—eyes, ears, nose, mouth and skin—are continually sampling the environment and forwarding data to my brain for processing. With the exception of our skin, the sense organs are in close physical proximity to the brain to shorten the transmission time, since we don't see, hear, smell, taste, or feel anything until the brain decodes what the senses detect.

Moving three times every second, my eyes shift rapidly from Janet's face to the pattern in her shirt, from the painting on the wall behind her to the floral arrangement on the table and back to Janet's face. It seems to me that I am seeing all these things simultaneously, but that is an illusion created by my brain. With each shift of my eyes, I clearly see about one percent of my surroundings while my brain fills in the missing bits.[1] My brain relies on what it just saw—plus assumptions based on past experiences—to fabricate a complete image of my surroundings in my mind. When my eyes focus on Janet's face, for example, my brain continues to show me that there are flowers on the table and a painting above her head because it remembers seeing those objects earlier. These objects in my peripheral vision appear hazy and indistinct, but they jump into focus as soon as I turn my attention toward them.

My relaxed scanning of Janet and our environment indicates that my nervous system is in the "rest, digest, and heal" state of homeostasis that we learned about earlier. But even in my relaxed state, my awareness is limited. To perceive every sight, sound, and scent in the environment would require more neural processing power than my brain possesses. So, it prioritizes incoming sensory data using selection criteria that researchers are still trying to understand. Scientists estimate that as much as 90 percent of the data collected by our eyes is ignored by the brain. The term "inattentional blindness" refers to our ability to look right at something (like an approaching vehicle) and not register its presence because our brain has chosen to ignore the visual input.[2] If you have ever searched for a lost item only to find it in a place you already checked, you have experienced inattentional blindness firsthand.

On the flip side, we might see something that is not actually present because our brain expects it to be there. If you ask me later, I might recall seeing a saltshaker on the table even if there wasn't one. It may be difficult to believe that our brain is showing us a manufactured image of our surroundings, but if there is sensory data that your brain is ignoring, how could you possibly know?

Suddenly my ears detect a sound nearby. My brain suspects it's a burst of laughter from diners at the next table, and it turns my head so my eyes can confirm its interpretation. At that exact moment, a metallic clatter emanates from the kitchen but—distracted by the nearby laughter—my brain ignores the commotion although Janet's brain hears it.

Not only am I sensing my environment with my five sense organs, but my sixth sense is also engaged. As we discovered earlier, we are miniature radio stations broadcasting and receiving emotional signals. When the door to the restaurant swings open, my attention shifts to the man who just entered. Something about his demeanor seems agitated, so he dominates my focus. With my attention on the man near the door, I don't notice that Janet is frowning at the boisterous table next to us.

Our survival instinct wields a powerful influence over us. A part of our focus is autonomic, meaning that we cannot consciously control it. Our brain is always asking, "Am I safe?" like a computer program running in the background. This is why the brain prioritizes incoming data that may signal a threat to our safety. When I detect agitated vibes from the man by the door, my casual scanning stops. My attention fixates on him while my brain is poised to activate the stress response. During those few seconds, my pupils dilate to let in more light, my heart beats a tiny bit faster, and my brain ignores incoming sensory data from other sources. As long as we feel safe, we engage in relaxed scanning of our surroundings. If we detect a potential threat, however, our attention locks in on it until our sense of security is restored. As soon as I realize that the man by the door is just picking up a takeout order, my attention shifts back to Janet.

Although Janet and I are enjoying lunch together at the same table, engaging in mutual conversation, we are each having a unique experience because we are focused on different things. Later, each of us will recall moments from our lunch together that the other failed to notice.

It is only natural that our memories of an event may differ from the memories of other people who experienced it with us. Janet's recollections of our lunch are just as valid as mine, even though we will each remember it differently. While it is reassuring when other people agree with us, we save ourselves a lot of unnecessary frustration when we acknowledge that all of us are experiencing our own unique reality. Arguing with others over the "reality" of a situation disrupts the flow of our biofield and lowers our vibe.

When we are caught up in the throes of chronic anxiety, our brain is constantly on high alert. It is more likely to interpret harmless people, comments, and situations as possible threats. As we fixate our flashlight of focus on one potential risk after another, the important aspects of our life recede into the hazy dark shadows beyond the beam. But it doesn't have to be that way. As you commit to practicing the techniques you have learned so far in this book, you will build resilience to stress, raise your vibe, and master the ability to direct your attention toward what matters most in your life.

Through the Eyes of Another

I was dining al fresco with a friend one day when suddenly a teensy spider appeared on the picnic table in front of me. This spider had two gorgeous spots of iridescent green on its face. Later, I discovered that it was a Bold Jumper, or *Phidippus audax*. When I exclaimed in delight at the beautiful colors sparkling in the sunlight, that spider cocked its head to peer up at me with its eight round eyes. I try to imagine what the spider saw when it gazed at my face. What does the world look like to a spider with 360-degree vision? If I could see myself through the spider's eyes, would I even recognize myself? Although I can pretend that the way I see the world is the "right" way and the spider's multi-eyed perspective is skewed, what if it's really the other way round? Perhaps you and I agree that a car is red, but does that mean that we both see the color red in the same way?

My cat Maxx and I have very different perspectives of the house that we live in together. With his eyes about nine inches above the floor, Maxx's world is full of legs—chair legs and human legs. His happy places include the highest perch on the cat tree and the cat bed under my desk. From my elevated vantage point, I have a distant relationship with legs of any kind. Spending time in my happy place does not involve climbing up the cat tree or scooching under the desk. Scientists tell us that humans and cats see light differently, so—if Maxx cared enough—we could have a spirited discussion about the color of the bedspread. While I need to switch on a lamp at night, his lowlight vision allows him to maneuver easily in the dark. And while Maxx needs a quick sniff to identify our other cat, Luna, I rely on my eyes to know when she walks into the room. When I pick Maxx up, his furry head swivels in wonder at this fresh perspective. It reminds me of the scene from *Dead Poet's Society* when the teacher, played by Robin Williams, urges his students to stand on their desks to see the classroom in a different way.

Intentional focus reminds us that we can choose how we view other people and situations. As humans, we have access to metacognition—the ability to think about our thinking. This allows us to widen our worldview and try to see things from the perspective of another. With practice, we can try to view political topics from perspectives that are the polar opposite of ours—although I wouldn't recommend starting there. Begin by seeing the world through the eyes of a spider or a cat. Imagine how limited our plodding two-eyed existence would seem to a tiny eight-eyed spider that can easily leap several feet. Consider how the room looks to Maxx from his perch at the top of the cat tree. Stand on your furniture or lie on the floor. When we try to see situations from another's perspective it can help us appreciate that there is more than one correct way to look at things.

It can be quite freeing to bring this level of flexibility to understanding the perceptions of other people. We can appreciate the validity of other perspectives even if we don't share them. We can relinquish our need for other people to agree with us.

While it garners a lot of media attention, the animosity expressed on social media is nothing new. Throughout human history, the unwillingness to recognize diverse perspectives has led to bloodshed. Practicing seeing the house from Maxx's viewpoint helps me accept that my reality is uniquely my own. It would be comical to insist that Maxx adopt my way of seeing things, don't you agree?

Can you think of a situation in which shifting your focus to the perspective of another might be beneficial?

The Energetic Currency of Focus

We spend part of our income on essentials such as food, housing, and transportation—the fundamental costs of living in our society. The rest of our income we spend on discretionary items—things we can choose to spend our money on such as entertainment.

In the last chapter, we discovered that everything is energy. There's a saying that "energy flows where attention goes."

Think of your focus like energetic currency. Whatever is illuminated in the beam of our flashlight of focus receives some of our energetic resources like a debit card withdrawal from our bank account. Our brain autonomously spends some of our focus monitoring our environment for threats. We choose (perhaps subconsciously) how we invest the discretionary portion of our energetic currency.

As I shared earlier, stressed-out old me was a pro at spinning up a tornado of self-induced stress every morning. As I went through the motions of getting ready for the day, internally I watched home movies on the screen of my imagination. Perhaps I had a presentation to upper management scheduled for that day. In my mind, I envisioned the opening slides and practiced what I would say.

Although mental rehearsal is an effective technique for enhancing performance, I allowed the scene to unfold from a negative slant. Instead of picturing a successful meeting, I imagined myself tripped up by questions I hadn't anticipated. Then my focus shifted from the future to the past as I recalled previous presentations derailed by the executive who regularly raised improbable objections that I had to defuse while suppressing the urge to scoff.

"What outlandish objection might get raised today, and how will I respond?" I wondered to myself. My heart pounded and my stomach clenched in response. A key step in my healing journey was listening objectively to my inner monologue. I realized that most of the time I was either imagining future problems or reliving unpleasant memories from the past. I was wasting my energetic currency.

Worrying about a past situation that we cannot change or a future situation that we cannot control (and may never actually happen anyway) is a waste of our valuable discretionary energy, comparable to throwing money into a bonfire. Regularly poking at old bruises from situations that I wished I had handled differently or imagining worst-case scenarios coming true only fueled my chronic anxiety, lowered my vibe, and exacerbated my health challenges.

The observer effect states that the act of paying attention to something changes it. McTaggart takes this into account in her peace intention experiments, by not revealing the geographical location to participants before the intention session. Otherwise, the energy of their attention could initiate changes in advance, thereby skewing the before and after comparison of violent crime in the area.

Intentional focus is about noticing what is illuminated by the beam of our attention. Are we investing discretionary attention toward a future where all our dreams come true? Or are we dwelling on unhealthful thoughts and emotions?

While I am not proposing ignoring the inevitable difficulties in life, we do not need to waste our energetic currency mulling over things we cannot change or control. Nor do we need to engage in debate with others over conflicting memories of a shared experience. It is highly unlikely—if not impossible—to argue someone else into trading their recollections for yours. These activities only deplete our energetic resources unnecessarily.

Instead, we can invest our energetic currency wisely by focusing on solutions versus problems. When we train ourselves to let go of thoughts that rob energy from "rest, digest, and heal" functions, we raise our vibration and optimize our health.

How are you spending your energetic currency?

Meet Scenario Sally

At first, whenever I caught myself straying into the movie theater of worries and regrets, I would shout at myself, "STOP! You are making this up!" That tactic worked very well, but over time I changed my approach.

As I asked myself why I was wasting my energetic currency, I realized that my home movies were just another aspect of our universal survival instinct. My mind was trying to protect me by rehearsing how I would shield myself if the worst were to happen. It was calling forth past "threatening" situations to try to learn from them. Having a defense strategy makes sense on the battlefield or the basketball court, but perhaps not so much in workplace situations such as giving a presentation. There is value in mentally and emotionally preparing ourselves for potentially tense situations. But when I allowed my mental rehearsal to escalate into a stress response, I lost connection with the part of my brain that could help me strategize creative solutions to those "what if" possibilities.

So, I made friends with my inner movie producer. I call her "Scenario Sally," because she is always acting out various scenarios like an actor rehearsing the delivery of her lines. I appreciate having Sally around (although I doubt that I could evict her even if I wanted to). If she gets too carried away with the drama of a situation, I holler, "Cut! Sally, you are overreacting." Or, when she revives scenes from the past, I tell her that there's no point looking back. It's easier for me to extract myself from the movie theater in my mind when I redirect my focus toward something else—such as my blessings.

The Benefits of a Gratitude Practice

What image comes to mind if I tell you not to think of a pink elephant? You just thought of one—am I right? When we try to suppress thoughts of something, it can have the opposite effect of pointing our flashlight beam directly at it. Instead of resisting a thought, embrace an alternative one by pointing your flashlight in another direction. This is where your list of what's important to you comes in handy. Practicing "in the moment" gratitude helps, as well.

When asked what we are grateful for, most of us list the big-ticket items: health, relationships, financial security, yada yada yada. While those things certainly deserve some of our intentional focus, I am going to challenge you to discover the smaller blessings in every moment.

When you find yourself in the theater of worries and regrets —dreading the future or regretting the past—take a deep breath and give thanks for whatever you are doing in the moment. If you are getting dressed, give thanks for your closet full of clean clothes. If you are walking into work, give thanks for your job. If you are doing household chores, give thanks for your house. Everything that we touch in our daily activities is not available to someone—safe drinking water, indoor plumbing, nourishing food, self-help books… The list is endless.

Gratitude is a high-vibe emotion that raises our frequency. Take a moment to look around you and notice at least five things that you are grateful for right now, at this moment. There's more to a gratitude practice than just thinking about those things; it is essential that we also feel the emotion of gratitude. I find it helpful to imagine for a moment what life would be like without the object of my gratitude. Then I experience a rush of joy that it is in my life.

Remember that the amplitude of the heart is greater than that of the brain. As you focus on the objects of your gratitude, direct your attention to the area of your heart chakra. Imagine it glowing with the frequency of gratitude. When I visualize heart chakra energy, I see pink, green and/or white light spiraling outward from the center of my sternum in front of and behind me.

Gratitude is such a nourishing practice that I begin every day experiencing it. When I open my eyes in the morning, I take a moment to shine my focus around the room. I consider all the refugees fleeing violence so that I really mean it when I think, "Thank you for this comfortable bed. I am happy to be in a place where I feel safe and secure." I send love to the roof over my head and the system that keeps my bedroom cool in the summer and warm in the winter. My fondness for indoor plumbing is deep and abiding regardless of the season, as I remember that outhouses were prevalent just a few generations ago.

As I sip my coffee, I recall the days when a work crisis would have deprived me of grabbing a cup in the morning. How lucky we are! I have running water at the twist of a knob, but my grandmother's farmhouse was equipped with a manual pump outside the kitchen door, which must have seemed a luxury to her parents because it eliminated the need to carry water from the spring behind the house. Doing household chores like laundry can be pleasurable when we remember that some people do not have access to clean clothes. Even when life doesn't go the way we would like, we can feel grateful for the opportunity to grow.

As we radiate high-vibe emotions like gratitude, we reap all the health benefits associated with "rest, digest, and heal." When we feel safe and calm, our awareness opens to the simple pleasures in every moment—the smell of a steaming cup of coffee, the softness of a cozy sweater, the pleasing sensations of a full belly, a text from a friend, warm sun on our skin—revealing even more reasons to feel grateful. With the rational brain fully online, we can tap into our creative problem-solving. Tasks that once appeared daunting seem more manageable.

Just as sunlight helps plants to grow, our flashlight of focus nourishes the important things in our lives. Direct the beam toward your gifts and watch them expand while your worries wither in the darkness. The flashlight is in your hands, and only you can choose where to shine your light.

Show Me Something Good

Have you heard the parable of the farmer? One day, the farmer's horse ran away. His neighbor came to commiserate with him. "How terrible that you lost your horse," exclaimed the neighbor. "How will you plow your fields in the spring?"

"Who knows if it is good or bad?" replied the farmer.

A week later, the farmer's horse returned followed by five strong, wild horses. His neighbor came to celebrate with him. "How fortunate that you now have six horses," declared the neighbor.

"Who knows if it is good or bad?" replied the farmer.

A week later, the farmer's son was attempting to train one of the strong, wild horses when it threw him off and broke his leg. The neighbor came to console him. "How awful that your son broke his leg," exclaimed the neighbor. "How will you manage to tend to the farm without your son's help?"

"Who knows if it is good or bad?" replied the farmer.

A week later, the army came through the countryside conscripting all the young men to go off to war, but they left the farmer's son behind due to his broken leg. His neighbor came to congratulate him. "How lucky that your son was not taken away," declared the neighbor.

"Who knows if it is good or bad?" replied the farmer.

As Shakespeare writes in Hamlet, "There is nothing either good or bad, but thinking makes it so." For me, the parable of the farmer is a reminder that there are both good and bad aspects to everything. Even if you hate your job and are actively seeking another one, you can find positive aspects to your current employment situation if you look for them. You can feel grateful for the income that you continue to receive until you find a job that you like better. You can also feel gratitude for the freedom to search for another job. Before cars and the internet, people's job opportunities were limited to employers in their physical vicinity. During the Industrial Age, people were forced to relocate to neighborhoods near the factories. When my grandmother graduated from college, being a nurse or schoolteacher were the only "acceptable" positions for an unmarried woman her age. As the yin yang symbol reminds us, everything has a dark and a light side to it.

Remember that we can choose whether to shine our flashlight of focus at the aspects of life that raise our vibe, or we can dwell on the aspects that elicit low-vibe emotions. When Scenario Sally takes the stage, instead of watching her act out a scene that I want to avoid, I say to her, "Thanks for the warning. Now, show me something good. Let's focus on the best-case outcome instead."

Finding Our Blind Spots

As my lunch with Janet illustrates, we cannot notice every aspect of our environment. Our senses detect what they detect, and our brain autonomically decides which sensory data to decode and which data to discard. What we perceive in our peripheral vision is a version of reality constructed by our brain as it sifts through and sorts incoming data and fills in missing bits with assumptions based on past experience. To see something clearly, we have to intentionally focus our attention on it.

The mechanics of eyesight are a metaphor for how we see the world. My first visit home from college was disorienting. My experiences that first semester—partying, staying out all night, losing my virginity—had changed me so much that I felt like a stranger in the home that I had left only a few months earlier. But my family only saw the me they remembered. No one focused closely enough to realize that the person I used to be was not there anymore.

There's a saying attributed to the Greek philosopher Heraclitus that you can never step in the same river twice. The molecules of water in a river are in a constant state of flux, as is the energy flowing through our biofield. The next time you are with a friend, colleague, or family member, intentionally focus on them. How have they changed since the last time you were together? Look past their outward appearance and note their energetic frequency. What emotions are prevalent in their field?

Not only is our sense of sight dependent on what the brain chooses to see, but our eyes have a literal blind spot. Light reflecting off the retina in each eye is transmitted to the brain via the optic nerve. The human eye has a blind spot due to a lack of photoreceptors where the optic nerve connects to the retina. When both eyes are open, the overlapping fields of view allow the brain to fill in the missing bits.

With one eye closed, however, the Blind Spot Test allows us to "see" this area of non-seeing. Using a black felt-tip marker, make a large dot on the left side of an index card and an "X" on the right side. Holding the card at arm's length with the "X" on the right side, close your right eye. Although you can see both symbols, focus your left eye on the "X" while slowly drawing the card toward you. The dot will disappear when the light reflecting off the dot aligns with the blind spot in your left eye. Next, close the left eye and focus your right eye on the dot. Bring the card closer until the "X" disappears.

We have virtual blind spots, as well. Our beliefs and past experiences blend together to form our personal version of reality. Then we seek out evidence to reinforce our perspective while discarding information that contradicts our worldview like an errant puzzle piece. This confirmation bias happens autonomically, similar to the brain choosing which visual data to decode and which to discard. We fool ourselves into believing that we are being realistic about a situation, blissfully unaware of what we are subconsciously choosing to ignore. We may rail about the injustice of another's actions without seeing how our behavior contributed to the situation. Or we may idealize someone or something while overlooking flaws that are obvious to others.

Our manufactured view of reality is not a character flaw. It is simply how we humans make sense of a complicated world of overwhelming and conflicting input. Situations that trigger our stress response or ignite strong emotions are the hardest to see clearly. One way to identify our blind spots is to pay attention to opinions that differ from our own. We can ask ourselves, "What are they seeing that I am not?"

Another method to reveal our blind spots is to play devil's advocate. Imagine what an opponent might say to convince us that we are wrong. Just as with Maxx and the spider, imagining a situation through the eyes of another loosens emotional barriers to clear-eyed discernment.

Old me was susceptible to righteous indignation, an intense anger directed at anything I deemed morally inappropriate. In addition to all the symptoms of an over-the-top "fight or flight" response, I felt as if my feet were stuck in concrete. I dug in my heels, convinced that my anger was justified. Do you ever feel that way? What I failed to understand at the time was the energetic cost of the associated stress, low vibes, and distraction from the important things in my life.

On top of that, anger accomplishes nothing and interferes with our creative problem-solving ability. With the benefit of hindsight, I can see that my blind spots and unwillingness to view situations from other perspectives fueled my righteous indignation. Now, when I sense righteous indignation creeping in, I concentrate on softening my heart. I remind myself that we are all imperfect beings and radiate unconditional love to the source of my ire.

Keep in mind that any information we receive from others is subject to their blind spots. Your friend may relate an alarming story of an argument with her boss while omitting the fact that the boss was upset because she dropped the ball on an important work assignment. A pundit may inflame their audience with stories of political ineptitude but fail to mention the bipartisan bills that recently passed. The content of every news story and book is subject to the inattentional blindness, confirmation bias, and blind spots of its creator. Remember that there is always more to the story than what we think we know about it.

The Tracing Infinity Technique

The infinity symbol—also referred to as the figure eight or *lemniscate* in geometry—appears in many healing systems, including tai chi and qigong. Composed of two interconnecting loops, the infinity symbol represents a closed system of constant movement, like the rivers of energy that flow through our meridians, our chakras, and throughout our entire energy field. Viewed from any angle, the loops are the same size, representing balance—front and back, side to side. As in the yin yang symbol, the infinity sign represents an indivisible whole of seemingly opposite forces of light and dark, like the farmer who could see each experience as either good or bad.

The Tracing Infinity Technique releases stuck energy associated with righteous indignation and can be useful whenever you feel emotional rigidity. This simple movement relaxes the muscles around the eyes, stimulates energy flow between the two hemispheres of the brain, quiets a busy mind, and stimulates a sense of peace and calm. I use it if I'm having trouble falling asleep.

This technique can be used anywhere on your body. During a healing session, sometimes I will trace infinity around my client's entire body from head to feet, crossing at the heart chakra. Try tracing the infinity symbol above a wound, an injury, or painful area to promote localized healing. Even repeatedly drawing the infinity symbol on a piece of paper has been shown to promote calm focus.

1. Begin with the Intentional Grounding Technique, which includes a few moments of Intentional Breathing.
2. Moving very slowly, use one or two fingers to trace a circle around one eye starting at the bridge of the nose a few inches away from your body.
3. Return to the starting point on the bridge of the nose and trace a circle around the other eye as if you are drawing the infinity sign on your face.
4. Repeat the process until you feel relaxed.

How to Direct Your Focus

In this chapter, we learned that our attention is a form of energetic currency. Intentional focus involves directing our energy toward what is most important in our life. Due to neurological limitations, we only perceive a portion of our surroundings. To see something clearly, we must focus on it. Our brain chooses what to pay attention to and fills in the blanks. This is why two people engaged in a shared activity will each have their own unique—yet equally authentic—experience.

Chronic anxiety redirects our energy into constantly scanning for threats and anticipating worst-case scenarios because stress makes us question our safety. The mechanics of eyesight also apply to the shaping of our beliefs and opinions. Confirmation bias and blind spots lead us to ignore information that conflicts with our worldview.

Here are some tips for directing your focus toward what is important:

1. Write this chapter's intention (*I intend to focus on what is important*) on a piece of paper and tape it to your bathroom mirror. Take a moment every morning to decide how you will practice the intention in the day ahead. At the end of the day, congratulate yourself for taking action to cultivate your personal power.
2. Intentional focus starts with paying attention to your thoughts. As you move through the rest of your day, notice (without judgement) where your flashlight is pointing and how it makes you feel.
3. Make a list of what is important to you and place it where you will see it every day. At the end of every day, estimate how much energetic currency you invested in what is important to you.
4. Pick a point in your existing daily routine to focus on the frequency of gratitude for two minutes at least twice every day. Use the Technique Practice Tracker in the back of the book to track your progress until it becomes a habit.
5. Recognize when the stress response is stealing your focus. Use Intentional Breathing and Tracing Infinity to restore a sense of calm.
6. Notice your inner dialogue. When it strays into the territory of future worries or past regrets, redirect your attention in a healthful direction using the Focuser Technique or practicing gratitude.

7. Avoid the temptation to dispute the memories, perceptions, and opinions of others. Remember that we each experience our own unique version of reality. There's no point trying to convince my cat Maxx that his view of our home is misinformed.
8. Exploring opinions that differ from ours can raise our awareness of our blind spots.
9. Retake the Chronic Anxiety Self-Assessment. Log your score in the Self-Assessment Tracker to monitor changes in your stress level over time.
10. Remember that your flashlight of focus is in your hands and only you can decide where to direct it.

SEVEN
INTENTIONAL MINDSET

I intend to adopt a growth mindset.

OUR MINDSET IS the lens through which we view ourselves and everything around us. It shapes our worldview, guides our decision-making, and influences our behavior. Do we view the world as safe or threatening? Do we choose the path of least resistance or pursue challenging goals? Do we give up easily or continue striving in the face of obstacles? As Henry Ford said, "Whether you believe you can, or you believe you can't—you're right."

Our mindset also wields a powerful influence over our physical, mental and emotional health. Since all healing is self-healing, our faith in our ability to heal influences whether we get better or not.

In the last chapter, we learned that all of us are experiencing our own unique reality, which is determined by where we direct the energetic currency of our focus. Our virtual blind spots may lead us to ignore information that doesn't fit with our worldview.

In this chapter, we will discover how our worldview was created in the first place and how it evolves. We will see that our perceptions of ourselves, other people, and the world around us directly affects our physical, mental, and emotional health.

American psychologist Carol Dwek, Ph.D., coined the term "growth mindset" to describe people who strive to constantly examine and evolve their mindset. Adopting a growth mindset involves asking ourselves, "*Why* do I think *what* I think?"

Our Mindset Affects Our Health

Hotel housekeepers scrub bathrooms, change bed linens, empty waste bins, vacuum rooms and hallways, and haul dirty sheets and towels to the hotel laundry. It's a physically demanding job that requires constant walking, bending, and lifting.

In 2007, a team of Harvard researchers led by mindfulness expert Dr. Ellen Langer conducted one of several studies to assess whether our mindset impacts us physiologically.[1] Considering that a housekeeper cleans fifteen rooms a day on average, it is interesting that when eighty-four hotel housekeepers were questioned, 66 percent reported that they did not exercise regularly. In their minds, exercise required lacing up running shoes or going to a gym.

At the outset of the study, the researchers collected baseline health data from the participants including:

- Weight
- Blood pressure
- Waist-to-hip ratio
- Body mass index
- Percent body fat (using bioelectrical impedance analysis)

They questioned the housekeepers about their health habits,

such as what they ate, their consumption of sugar, caffeine, and alcohol, their nicotine use, and their perceived amount of exercise.

Then the researchers told half of the participants (the Informed Group) that the movement required by their job exceeded the CDC's recommendations for an active lifestyle. Participants were given handouts showing the estimated caloric expenditure for various cleaning tasks. Housekeepers at the other hotels (the Control Group) were only told they would get health improvement feedback at the conclusion of the study.

Over the next four weeks, management at each hotel ensured that the participants' workload stayed steady. In other words, all the participants maintained the same activity level at work. Their health habits remained consistent, too. No surprise there—we all know how difficult it can be to change eating habits or give up nicotine, alcohol, caffeine, or sugar.

Although the Informed Group did not change their physical activity level, their perception of exercising regularly doubled—because they now viewed their work tasks as exercise. The Informed Group experienced significant improvements in every physiological measure. Mean weight dropped nearly two pounds. Mean blood pressure dropped from 130/80 to 120/75. Keep in mind—this is over a four-week period, and nothing changed except the participants' mindset.

The authors of the study concluded that our beliefs have a measurable effect on our physical reality. As the study states, "... It is time for all of us to explore more direct means of controlling our health, such as pursuing mindfulness as a tool to actively and deliberately change our mind-sets."

If you are feeling skeptical, this is just one study showing that our physical body changes based on what we believe. In a separate experiment, a research team at Yale University invited participants to taste-test milkshakes that they were told would be given to patients in the hospital. Two taste tests were conducted a week apart. The label on one shake touted its sensible low-fat healthiness, while the other shake was labeled "high fat" and "indulgent." Not only did people report that the indulgent shake was more satisfying, but the levels of ghrelin (a hunger hormone) in their bloodstream dropped significantly after ingesting what they believed was the high-fat shake. By now, you may have guessed that both milkshakes were exactly the same—yet their *belief* that one shake provided more calories affected their body in a measurable, though autonomic, way.

In a study out of Japan, researchers told participants that they were rubbing their arms with leaves from a plant similar to poison ivy. Even though the leaves were harmless, all thirteen participants had a reaction consistent with contact dermatitis.

In a 2013 study reported in the *New England Journal of Medicine*, patients diagnosed with a medial meniscus tear—a type of knee injury—experienced the same level of pain relief up to twelve months later regardless of whether they had arthroscopic surgery or sham surgery.[2] Their knee felt better even if all the doctor did was put them to sleep and make incisions without performing the full procedure.

These studies indicate that our mindset can have a powerful impact on our physical health, even going so far as to manipulate our blood hormone level and trigger a skin rash. But where does our mindset come from in the first place?

Making Up Our Mindset

When I was five years old, we lived in a small rural community. Dissatisfied with the inventory at the local market, my mom decided to shop for groceries in a larger store fifteen miles away. Impressed by the wide-open space, my preschool self commenced skipping up and down the aisles shouting out the names of the products I could identify: "Beans! Rice! Soup!" Too young to read, I skipped right past the "Wet Floor" sign and landed on the hard linoleum floor with a thump. Nursing a bruised bum and confined to the shopping cart in my now wet pants, I whimpered to go home while my embarrassed mom completed her shopping. I perked up at the register, however, eyeing the colorful array of candy bar wrappers. "You don't deserve a candy bar," hissed my exasperated mom. Her words left an impression on my young mind. Many years later, when my baby brother cried because my mom refused to buy him a toy, I informed my younger sibling in my best imitation of a grown-up voice, "You don't deserve a toy!"

Our mindset is shaped by our beliefs, values, personal experiences, social conditioning, our sense of self, and information from sources that we trust. Although these elements are tightly interwoven, we will explore each separately.

1. Don't Believe Everything You Think

Childhood is a time of firsts: our first tooth, first haircut, and first cup with a tight-fitting lid to prevent spills. It is also when we receive our starter kit of beliefs—facts we accept about ourselves and the world around us. Some of our beliefs support a healthful mindset, while others influence our behavior in ways that limit our personal growth.

Our brain stays in input mode until about age six. We are little sponges soaking up everything without discernment; as children, we lack the capability to question what we see and hear. Whatever people say is indiscriminately programmed into our psychic operating system. In the movie *The Help*, the character Aibileen repeatedly reminds the toddler Mae, "You is kind. You is smart. You is important." Aibileen understands the effect her words will have on Mae's self-esteem later in life.

Likewise, a disparaging remark from a frustrated parent, jealous sibling, or overworked teacher becomes a limiting belief that persists into adulthood. When my mom told me that I didn't deserve a treat, I created the belief that my worthiness depended on my behavior. While this belief may make it easier for a parent to manage their child when they are young, we can grow up to be non-assertive, people-pleasing perfectionists. To this day, I feel uncomfortable treating myself unless I believe I have done something to deserve it.

2. What's It Worth to You?

Our beliefs intersect with our values. For example, gratitude is a value rooted in the belief that we should express appreciation for our life circumstances. Values are often tied to morality, since they may influence our sense of right and wrong behavior.

We are more likely to bond with people who share our values. I value honesty because I believe it is wrong to lie (probably because I got in huge trouble for lying as a child). For a brief time, I was friends with a woman named Lori. As we got to know each other, I learned that she had no reservations about lying to get what she wanted. Lori was comfortable with her misleading résumé because it landed her a position with a significant salary increase. "It's the recruiter's fault that they didn't bother to verify my credentials," she laughed.

Once, Lori told her boss she had a doctor's appointment so she could spend the afternoon shopping at a local boutique. "I didn't want to miss the sale," she explained. Lori, like the rulers Machiavelli described in his book *The Prince*, believed that the ends justified the means; as long as she achieved the desired results, it didn't matter how she got it. If Lori valued truthfulness, I doubt she would have spoken to me so openly about her deceptions. Needless to say, our friendship was short-lived because I couldn't respect Lori or trust anything she said to me.

Do you have someone like Lori in your life? One way to identify your values is to bring to mind people who tend to rub you the wrong way. There might be something about their behavior that violates your values.

3. What Happened to You?

As we mature, our mindset is influenced by our personal experience. For example, someone who achieves a prosperous lifestyle after laboring long hours for many years values hard work because—based on their first-hand experience—hard work pays off. On the other hand, someone who struggles to pay the bills despite working multiple jobs may not value hard work because it has not brought them prosperity. Both perspectives are valid despite being polar opposites. Hard work *can* pay off, but it doesn't *always*.

When we feel hurt or angry, the issue is not the situation itself but the meaning we assign to it. Perhaps at some point Lori had suffered for speaking truthfully, so she decided that honesty was not the best policy for her. As the Buddha taught, situations are neutral. It is us who interpret a situation as positive or negative; something we wish to prolong or something we wish to avoid.

4. Where Did You Come From?

Expectations of our tribe concerning acceptable dress, food, behavior, and relationships with others also influence our mindset. Talking during a movie or play violates my expectations of acceptable behavior, but plenty of people feel comfortable doing it. When I first began visiting a family from the Middle East, I would brush aside the proffered cup of tea because I didn't want to inconvenience them (plus, I hadn't earned it), but when I learned that declining tea is rude in their culture, I accepted with gratitude.

Often our concepts regarding gender identity originate from social conditioning—for example, the respective roles assigned to men and women, the division of labor between our parents, the colors we wore as children, and the toys we played with.

What behaviors might lead to someone being ousted from

your tribe? Once in a business meeting, I observed two people from New York City lob criticisms at each other that I considered shockingly offensive. In my experience, that behavior could have serious consequences. But after the meeting adjourned, they chatted amiably and even made plans to meet up for dinner later. The experience prompted me to question whether New Yorkers lack proper manners or whether I, having been raised in the South, was overly demure. I realized that sometimes I refrain from saying what I think because—according to my upbringing—it could be perceived as rude.

5. Who Are You?

Often, we create our sense of self based on our understanding of feedback received from our family, friends, and society at large. If your parents constantly referred to you as their outgoing child, for example, that might continue to influence how you see yourself.

Our social conditioning can play a major role in shaping our sense of self. Because I grew up surrounded by makers, I have always felt comfortable engaging in activities such as drawing, painting, photography, sewing, and knitting. I believe that everyone is creative in some way. Perhaps their artistry lies in cooking, verbal expression, or how they dress. But my friend Margaret, a certified public accountant, strenuously objects when I encourage her to explore her creative side. "I'm not an artist," she repeatedly insists. According to Julia Cameron, author of *The Artist's Way*, some parents squash their child's creative tendencies to protect them from what they perceive as frivolous pursuits. Could something similar have happened to Margaret?

Ironically, we are more likely to notice (and criticize) other people for exhibiting qualities we dislike in ourselves. Research from 2022 revealed that participants were more likely to judge other people's bodies if they were dissatisfied with their own.

Even after losing weight, I still feel uncomfortable around people who wear tight shirts over their poochy bellies because I was self-conscious of my own tummy size.

How we feel about ourselves impacts the flow and vibration of our energy. My client Kai was struggling with persistent elbow pain. I noticed that Kai was quick to openly criticize himself. He would say things like, "I never learn" or "I have a mind like a sieve." Sensing that he would benefit from some self-love, I suggested that Kai send love to his elbow. He told me that was impossible, because he hated his elbow for disrupting his daily activities. When we say mean things about ourselves, we create pools of energetic congestion in our body. Unfortunately, Kai continued to struggle with elbow pain even after undergoing corrective surgery.

We can enhance our self-identity by focusing on the aspects of ourselves that we are proud of. Even if there is something about ourselves that we are working to change, we can accept ourselves as we are now. Loving ourselves unconditionally reduces stress, raises our vibe, and promotes self-healing. Plus, I believe that we can't love others until we love ourselves.

Above all, avoid comparing yourself to others. Envy is a low-vibe emotion. Remember that none of us is enjoying a carefree life regardless of outward appearances. Celebrate your special uniqueness!

6. Who Do You Trust?

A 2013 study concluded that patients are more likely to trust the competency of a medical professional wearing a white lab coat as opposed to scrubs or other attire.[3] In the studies mentioned earlier, participants trusted the researchers who told them that the milkshakes were different and that the leaves would cause a rash.

Information from sources that we trust influences what we

believe to be true. According to a 2024 article from the Pew Research Center, adults under the age of thirty trust information from social media nearly as much as they trust national news reports.[4] Whatever news source you rely on, it probably presents information in a way that is consistent with your beliefs, values, and other aspects of your mindset.

Since we can rarely travel to the site of current events to observe them ourselves, it is critical to keep in mind that reporters also contend with blind spots and confirmation bias. Even a firsthand account from a trustworthy friend is subject to what their brain chose to notice, just like my experience at lunch with Janet when I failed to hear the clatter from the kitchen.

Pay attention to how competing news sources spin the stories. Often, the words they choose subtly convey an opinion. For instance, referring to someone as "the accused" implies the possibility of innocence, while "the perpetrator" suggests guilt. One person's "freedom fighters" are someone else's "rebels" or even "terrorists."

Be wary, too, of getting all your information from one place. Seeking out news from disparate sources will make it easier to discern the facts from the opinions.

EACH OF THESE mindset components are interrelated. For example, if we see ourselves as capable and deserving of success (self-identity), we are more likely to find that hard work pays off (personal experience) because we embrace persistence (value) and keep striving until it does (behavior). When her boss introduced a creative team-building exercise, Margaret was uncomfortable participating (behavior) because she saw herself as analytical (self-identity) and lacking artistic talent (belief).

The Mindset Map exercise in the back of the book (and the online companion) provides journal prompts to explore your personal mindset. Use the results to complete the Limiting

Beliefs exercise to unpack beliefs that may be limiting your personal growth.

Mark's Story

When Mark's cancer returned, he initially declined treatment because chemotherapy made him very sick the first time (personal experience), he doubted it would work since his cancer had come back (belief), and he prioritized the quality of his life over longevity (value). At eighty years old, Mark also believed that his years were numbered anyway. "I've lived a long life and am at peace with the inevitable," he told me. Another aspect of Mark's mindset was that conventional cancer treatment was his only option. After encouragement from family members, Mark agreed to undergo chemotherapy, but his "why" was more for them than for himself. When the tumors continued to grow, the doctor's prognosis that he had three months left to live came from a source that he trusted. Mark's mindset became his reality. Three months later—to the day—Mark took his last breath.

There are many accounts of people who reclaimed their health after refusing to accept a terminal prognosis. Common to these situations is the view that one can heal oneself (belief), a strong sense of autonomy (value), faith in one's abilities (self-identity) and a willingness to try complementary therapies (information from sources that are trusted).

Remember, as humans, we have the unique gift of metacognition—the ability to think about our thinking. Intentionally adopting a growth mindset means asking ourselves, "*Why* do I think *what* I think?" This is a practice best approached with an air of curiosity instead of criticism, since we began manufacturing our mindset at a very early age. Through intention, we can reshape our mindset by choosing to focus our attention on the beliefs and other mindset components that raise our vibe.

The Life Lesson Journaling Exercise

I believe that life experience is a steady stream of opportunities to learn and grow, but we have free will to either embrace or ignore the lessons. According to Cherie Carter-Scott's *12 Rules for Being Human:*[5]

> You will be given lessons.
> There are no mistakes, only lessons.
> A lesson will be repeated until it is learned.
> Learning lessons does not end.

We can begin to understand our mindset by examining behavior patterns that lower our vibe, waste our valuable focus, and stunt our personal growth. Often, these patterns fall into the category of finances or relationships. Perhaps you live paycheck to paycheck, struggling to pay off debts despite a well-paying job. Perhaps you quit one job to escape a domineering boss only to find yourself working for another one. Or maybe you repeatedly fall in love with someone who seems like the perfect partner, only to experience the same heartbreak every time. Disappointing situations that play out repeatedly in our lives may provide clues to how our mindset can be improved.

Journaling is my preferred method to excavate the lesson in problematic patterns of behavior. By forcing us to slow our thinking, writing can unlock insights that our rational mind may race past. Then we can use the neuroplasticity of our brain to abandon aspects of our mindset that no longer serve us and find our new truth.

In the last chapter, I said that dwelling on the past is a waste of energetic currency. This exercise is an exception, since we are revisiting past experiences explicitly to learn lessons that can help us avoid repeating destructive patterns.

There is a tendency to make ourselves the hero (or the victim) in our memories, but for this exercise to be effective we have to be brutally honest with ourselves. If you are worried about someone reading what you wrote, use scrap paper and throw it away afterward.

1. Pick a time when you will have uninterrupted focus. Spend a few moments practicing the Focuser Technique.
2. Choose a behavior pattern that you wish to change. Write it down in the form of a question—for example, "How is my mindset contributing to my pattern of financial difficulties?" Or "How is my mindset contributing to my pattern of romantic breakups?"
3. Review your answers to the Mindset Map exercise, noting any beliefs, values, and so on that relate to your question.
4. Set a timer for ten minutes and start writing whatever comes into your head. When the timer goes off, read what you wrote out loud. Hearing the vibrations of your voice may unlock fresh realizations. If that happens, write those down as well.
5. What's the lesson you extracted from this exercise? Did you discover any "truths" you have been carrying around that may not be accurate? For example, I learned that my worthiness is not contingent on behaving in a way that pleases others.
6. How can you reframe your mindset? When my mom told me that I didn't deserve a treat due to my behavior in the grocery store, my child brain lacked the maturity to realize that she was not referring to my worthiness as a person. With the benefit of an adult perspective, I can try to look at the situation from Mom's perspective. We live in a society that judges parents' competency by the actions of their children. So, no doubt she was embarrassed by my behavior. We lived in a rural area where everyone knew everyone

> and, considering the limited options for groceries, we
> would be shopping at this store again. Mom was
> hoping to avoid a repeat of my behavior in the future.

This exercise can be challenging if your emotions are running high. If that happens, pick a future date to revisit the topic when you can approach it calmly.

Remember that you aren't perfect. Forgive yourself for things you did or said that you regret. Don't fret if you weren't able to unpack the lesson this time. Untangling our mindset can take time. At some future date, life will grant you another opportunity. After all, the lessons are repeated until they are learned.

How Stress Affects Our Mindset

As we learned earlier, chronic stress shifts our brain into survival mode, leading us to focus our attention on scanning for potential danger. Confirmation bias may cause us to discard information that indicates we are safe and latch onto perceived threats instead. As our vibe drops, our ability to think rationally is impeded. Fear makes us uncomfortable with uncertainty. We are desperate for an explanation that helps us make sense of our situation. We need to identify the source of danger, so we can defend ourselves.

The world's reaction to the COVID-19 pandemic illustrates what can happen to our mindset in extremely stressful situations. A highly dangerous virus had spread around the world. Hospitals erected makeshift wards to accommodate all the patients. The death toll rose daily. While scientists rushed to study the virus, we were uncertain who to trust in the ensuing hailstorm of conflicting information. We were being attacked by an invisible, life-threatening foe and had no idea how to defend ourselves. As a result, we became more susceptible to conspiracy theories, which typically offer a rationale for what is happening along with a villain to blame.

Popular conspiracy theories during COVID-19 blamed the Chinese government, incompetent medical experts, or a nefarious group of billionaires intent on taking over the world. A known attacker is less threatening than an unseen one. Conspiracy theories transform our fear into anger, which is a higher-vibe emotion. Having a target to blame can be so reassuring that we cling to a conspiracy theory even though it perpetuates the fight-or-flight response.

Cultivating resilience to stress makes us more comfortable with uncertainty and therefore less vulnerable to conspiracy theories. Techniques like Intentional Breathing and Grounding can dispel fear and raise our vibe. The Focuser and Infinity techniques can help us access the rational part of our brain for clearer thinking. The more we practice these techniques, the easier it will become for us to reclaim our calm following a stress response.

Reprogramming Through Affirmations

Just as the hotel housekeepers chose to view their work as exercise, we can improve our health by intentionally shifting our mindset. Changing our mindset involves identifying the old programming that is not serving us and then replacing it with a healthy belief. But even if we aren't consciously aware of those false beliefs, we can still reprogram our limiting beliefs through positive affirmations.

An affirmation is a statement of our desired future state, said as if the transformation has already occurred. For example, when I started my weight-loss journey, I would use the affirmation, "I am lean and healthy. Every molecule of my being is functioning perfectly." As I repeated this affirmation to myself, I conjured an image of myself at my ideal weight and moving with ease. Mentally scanning my body from head to foot, I pictured each cell performing optimally. I allowed myself to feel like I was already the future me. Although I have attained my weight-loss goal, I still practice this affirmation regularly. Every time, waves of gratitude and deep satisfaction flow through me.

I decided to recite my affirmations every time I walked up or down the stairs. At the time, I worked in a tall office building. When I entered or left the building, went to the cafeteria, or anytime I was only going a few floors up or down, I would use the stairwell instead of the elevator. Reciting my affirmations on the steps not only meant that I was revisiting my affirmations at least four times a day, but it also provided the added benefit of taking my mind off the effort of stair climbing.

A client once told me that affirmations are a form of "fake it until you make it," but I disagree. The attitude with which we practice our affirmations matters. Faking it implies that we are deceiving ourselves. When I recite an affirmation, I am setting an intention to evolve into an envisioned future self. Every day, we make choices that determine our future path. Affirmations remind us where we want to go so that we are more aware of whether those daily choices are moving us in the right direction. Affirmations are the North Star by which we navigate to our future dreams.

In the back of the book, and in the online companion, is an exercise to create your own personal list of affirmations.

Self-Defeating Programming

Many people would be surprised to learn that they already use affirmations. Their ongoing inner dialogue may sound something like this:

- I don't deserve anything better.
- I can't do this.
- The world is a dangerous place.
- Money is the root of all evil.
- Everyone is out to get me.

Without realizing it, they are using the power of affirmations to stay in the rut they profess they want to escape. They are reinforcing obstacles to their own transformation by justifying their limitations. When things don't change in their lives, it serves to reinforce their belief that attempts are futile, which becomes a self-fulfilling prophecy.

It is also possible to override affirmations. If I say to myself, "I am lean and healthy," but my inner critic retorts, "Are you kidding? Look at yourself!" I am neutralizing the affirmation by instantly reinstalling the same old programming. This is another reason why it is so important to pay attention to the voice in your head and not believe everything you think.

Observing our self-talk is one way to unearth those "truths" buried in the deep recesses of our brain. Listening to my inner monologue was perhaps the single most important step in my transformation journey.

Spend some time listening to your inner monologue. Is it kind or critical? Does it say things that build you up or tear you down? Does it express beliefs that serve you, or does it express outmoded ideas that warrant reprogramming? Make friends with your inner critic by acknowledging that it wants to protect you. Give your inner critic a name. Whenever it expresses low-vibe emotions like fear or anger, reassure it that everything is okay.

Remember that we are in charge of our thoughts and can choose how to interpret the situations in our life. Even entrenched beliefs can be overwritten if they are no longer serving us.

How to Evolve Your Mindset

In this chapter, we discovered how our mindset is the product of our beliefs, values, experiences, social conditioning, and information from sources that we trust. As our life unfolds, we can choose to evolve our mindset through fresh experiences and new information.

Our mindset affects how we see ourselves and the world around us. It not only influences our choices and behavior, but it also directly affects our physical, mental, and emotional health. Here are some tips for evolving your mindset:

1. Write this chapter's intention (*I intend to embrace a growth mindset*) on a piece of paper and tape it to your bathroom mirror. Take a moment every morning to decide how you will practice the intention in the day ahead. At the end of the day, congratulate yourself for taking action to cultivate your personal power.
2. Remember that you manufactured your mindset, which means that you have the power to change it. When someone's behavior bothers you, it may provide clues to your mindset. Their actions may be violating your values or beliefs. Use your journal to explore what the situation can teach you about yourself.
3. When life goes off track, ask yourself, "What is the lesson I can learn from this situation?" To break free from unhealthy patterns of behavior, examine how your beliefs, values, experiences, and social conditioning may be influencing your choices. Monitor your inner dialogue for self-criticism and make peace with your inner critic.
4. Use the Affirmations exercise to create a list of affirmations to reprogram your limiting beliefs. Practice reciting your affirmations twice a day for seven days. Use the Technique Practice Tracker in the back of the book to log your practice.
5. Continue to cultivate resilience to stress so you are better equipped to deal with uncertainty. Recognize that people latch onto conspiracy theories to restore a

sense of safety when confronting invisible foes. Try to respond compassionately.
6. Retake the Chronic Anxiety Self-Assessment. Log your score in the Self-Assessment Tracker to monitor changes in your stress level over time.
7. Make it a habit to ask yourself, *"Why* do I think *what* I think?"

EIGHT
INTENTIONAL RELEASE

I intend to release energetic blockages.

THERE'S A SAYING that to receive a gift, our hands must be empty. If our hands are grasping onto resentment, regret, resistance, or material items, then we are energetically stuck. With nothing going out, nothing new can come in—which leads to stagnation.

This chapter is about letting go. As you understand by now, stagnant biofield energy can lead to physical disease over time. Recall how choking back my frustration contributed to two frozen shoulders.

The premise behind HT and other energy medicine modalities is to clear these blockages so the body can heal itself. When a client's pain clears during an HT session—only to return again and again—it indicates that they may be burdened by past resentments or regrets. By focusing their attention on old wounds, they keep recreating the energetic blockages so that eventually the pain returns.

Just as painful memories contribute to energetic congestion, material objects can also weigh us down. Stuffing our homes with possessions is the energetic equivalent of walling ourselves off from the flow of new experiences.

Intentional release is about getting to the root of persistent energy blockages. We will examine the practice of forgiveness—for ourselves and for others—so we can release the past and move forward into our future. We will learn a journaling exercise to unearth unconscious burdens, and a powerful energy psychology technique for releasing stuck energy.

Wanda's Story

Wanda and I had been hiking for a few hours when we paused to rest in the shade of a pine grove. The sun was intense, but a gentle breeze made the heat bearable. As we chatted, Wanda steered the conversation toward the drama with her sister. I had heard this story many times before. Throughout the three years we had been friends, Wanda had nursed resentment toward her sister. She blamed her animosity on a disagreement over the settlement of their parents' estate, but my intuition told me there was more to the story.

The rift with her sister led to a fissure in the family. As a result, Wanda spent birthdays and holidays home alone.

Even though they hadn't spoken in years, Wanda invested significant time and energy grousing about her sister. As Wanda once again recounted the familiar story, her anger steadily grew. Instead of enjoying the pine-scented shade around us, Wanda was mired in a muddy swamp of resentment.

"I think you need to forgive your sister," I suggested. "You get angry at her on a regular basis, while she is off living her life. This anger is a burden that only hurts you."

Wanda looked at me with shocked disappointment. "Some things are unforgivable," she snapped.

Not long afterward, Wanda developed health issues that included excessive weight loss. Eventually, a large tumor was discovered in her lower colon. According to Louise Hay's book *You Can Heal Your Life*, health issues related to the colon may be caused by holding on to the past or a fear of letting go.[1] The tumor was close to the Root chakra—which, among other things, is associated with familial relationships and our sense of belonging. From the perspective of biofield health, Wanda's long-standing resentment toward her sister may have contributed to formation of the tumor.

Loading Up Our Burden Bags

Picture a hiker exploring the forest with a day pack containing essentials such as water, food, and maps. Many of us are hiking through life carrying a bag of energetic burdens—old wounds, regrets, resentments, past injustices; these are provisions that weigh us down as opposed to supporting us on our life journey. We keep our burden bag within easy reach so we can remove the contents regularly and examine them closely. We polish away the dust of time, renewing our righteous indignation with a fresh surge of adrenaline.

Why do we do that? Obviously, it would be better for our health to clear the pain from our biofield, restoring a healthy flow of electromagnetic energy.

One reason is to use our burden bag to distract us from darker underlying emotions. Low-frequency emotions such as shame, guilt, and fear are unpleasant, which is why we try to suppress them by reaching for a higher-vibe emotion such as anger. Wanda's intense focus on the injustice caused by her selfish sister could be a defense against acknowledging her own role in their damaged relationship. By focusing on her anger...an emotion with a frequency of 150 Hz, Wanda could be avoiding feelings of guilt...a much lower vibe emotion at 30 Hz. As Dr. David Hawkins points out in his book *Letting Go: The Pathway of Surrender*, "We typically feel so much guilt about anger that we find it necessary to make the object of our anger 'wrong' so that we can say our anger is justified."[2] Perhaps whenever Wanda misses her sister, renewing her anger alleviates her pain.

It takes a lot of energy, however, to ignore our feelings. Suppressed emotions cause energetic blockages that deplete our body's ability to fight infections, eliminate pre-cancerous cells, and replenish bones, blood, and muscle. In my experience, suppressing my anger toward my mother-in-law led to two frozen shoulders. Sara was able to quell her fear during the day, but as bedtime neared, she was too tired to contain it any longer, and it resulted in night terrors. Ironically, avoiding our feelings doesn't make them fade away. Instead, they lurk in the hazy shadows at the edges of our flashlight beam. As long as we don't look directly at them, we can pretend our low-vibe emotions don't exist, even as their energetic congestion festers in our biofield.

In his book *When the Body Says No,* physician Gabor Maté offers convincing evidence of the link between repressed emotions and conditions such as autoimmune diseases, cancer, digestive ailments, and diabetes. While Maté recognizes that genetics and toxins (like nicotine) play a role, not everyone with a BRAC gene mutation or cigarette habit will develop cancer. There must be other variables in the equation. He painstakingly detangles the emotional lives of his patients through introspective conversations, as well as interviews with family members, unearthing burdensome wounds from familial dysfunction and childhood trauma. Maté cautions, "When we have been prevented from learning how to say no, our bodies may end up saying it for us."[3] By educating us on the inexorable link between emotional and physical health, Maté is urging us to release blockages that could eventually make us sick.

Another reason for carrying our burdens with us is that we don't know *how* to let them go. A socially conditioned mindset that "boys don't cry" and "good girls are always nice" leaves us bereft of the tools we need to process our emotions in healthy ways. Experiencing anger does not mean storming about, shouting and smashing dishes. Instead, Maté advises transforming anger through validating the legitimacy of our emotions, exploring our emotional patterns and asserting healthy boundaries.

Hawkins states that our feelings naturally dissipate when we point our flashlight directly at them. "Letting go involves being aware of a feeling, letting it come up, staying with it, and letting it run its course without wanting to make it different or do anything about it. It means simply to let the feeling be there and to focus on letting out the energy behind it."[4]

There is an observable reaction when a client releases pent-up emotions during an HT session. Sometimes, there is a full-body twitch reminiscent of the *pop* when one squeezes bubble wrap. Crying or yawning are other indications that stuck energy has started to move. In HT sessions with animals, I have observed a deep sigh or shiver.

More subtly, you may feel airy as the load in your burden bag lightens. Your body feels limp as muscles go from contracted to relaxed. Colors may appear brighter. As the frequency of your vibration rises, things that used to irritate you feel irrelevant. You may feel awash in love for yourself and others.

The Burden Bag Release Exercise

Let's unpack your burden bag. We will use the Life Lesson Journaling Exercise from the last chapter, with a few tweaks.

Remember that we have a tendency to make ourselves the hero (or the victim) of our stories. For this exercise to be effective, though, we have to be brutally honest with ourselves. If you are worried about someone reading what you write, use scrap paper and throw it away afterward.

1. Pick a time when you will have uninterrupted focus. Spend a few moments practicing the Focuser Technique.

2. Ask yourself to consider what suppressed emotions might be lurking in your burden bag. If you frequently express righteous indignation, what situation or memory is associated with that emotion? Is there a past experience that you try to avoid remembering?
3. Write down the emotions that arise. Start with "I feel …" and list all the feelings that come up.
4. If you listed several emotions, choose one to examine first. Focus your attention on the feeling. Where do you feel it in your body? How does it feel? For example, is it cold, warm, or buzzy? How would you rate the intensity? Lean in to the sensations. Say out loud or to yourself, "It is safe for me to feel this way."
5. Put your hands on the part of your body where you feel the emotion—perhaps your head, chest, stomach, hips, or knees. Imagine white light flowing between your palms like a laser, clearing away stuck energy.
6. Stay with the emotion for as long as you can. Notice if it shifts or changes in intensity. Hawkins advises[5] that feelings typically run their course within twenty minutes.
7. When the emotion has dissipated or you need to take a break, journal about your experience. What insights did you gain?
8. If you listed more than one emotion in step three, repeat steps four through six with another emotion. You can do that now or come back to this exercise when you feel ready.

Remember that you aren't perfect. Forgive yourself for things you did or said that you regret. Don't fret if you weren't able to process all your emotions immediately. Some of us have been adding to our burden bag for years, and it will take time to unpack it all.

Pain is a Gift

If our hiker has an overloaded pack or hikes too far, their body will begin to protest. Their back may start to ache, or their calf muscle might constrict in an agonizing cramp. Our body speaks to us in sensations and pain is its way of getting our attention so we can stop what we are doing before we injure ourselves. Pain is a signal that it is time for the hiker to take a rest or reduce the weight in their pack before serious damage occurs.

Low-vibe thoughts and emotions can damage our body as surely as an overly strenuous hike. Recall my client Kai, who had the persistent elbow pain. Unwilling to send loving, healing energy to his elbow and convinced that HT could not help him, Kai resorted to surgery after just a few sessions. When surgery failed to alleviate his elbow pain, I sensed that the emotional burden of caring for his aging father was the root cause. It would not have been appropriate to express anger toward his father, so Kai aimed his frustration at his elbow instead. The physical pain was his body's way of letting Kai know that he needed to release his anger.

Remember my client Paul who had his left knee replaced? Paul had experienced knee pain before. The pain mysteriously disappeared for a few years, but when it returned, he elected to have surgery to remediate the pain once and for all.

At the time, Paul's boss had asked him to take over a dysfunctional team. Paul wanted to retire but continued working because he felt obligated to help his boss despite the elevated stress.

Flipping through Paul's medical records during his last appointment before the surgery, the doctor noticed that previously the pain had been in Paul's right knee. Undoubtedly, Paul's left knee was sufficiently compromised to justify joint replacement surgery—but recall that all healing is self-healing. Paul's right knee had healed on its own, so perhaps his left knee could have healed as well, once the work situation was addressed.

The next time you are struggling with physical pain, ask your body what it is trying to tell you. Is there a lesson lurking under the pain? Unexplained chronic pain can be frustrating, debilitating, and informative. Remember that pain can be a gift.

Practicing Forgiveness

I mulled over Wanda's words, "some things are unforgivable," for weeks. If she is correct, I reasoned, does that mean we are destined to carry certain burdens to the end of our days? Or can we choose to release our pain no matter how significant the transgression?

Practicing forgiveness is immensely freeing for me. Buried deep in the depths of my burden bag was shame from sexual abuse I experienced as a teenager. At 20 Hz, shame occupies the lowest rung on Hawkin's Map of Consciousness.[6] Rationally, I understood that what had happened to me wasn't my fault, but I still worried what people would think of me if they knew. When I learned that sexual abusers often were molested themselves, I had a flash of my abuser as a scared little boy while some adult committed atrocities against him. I'll never know if that really happened, but the possibility helped me find the compassion I needed to forgive him.

What does it mean to forgive? Forgiveness is a high-vibe emotion at a frequency between optimism and understanding. I believe forgiveness is a gift that we give ourselves by lightening our low-vibe emotional burdens. Releasing those emotions allows us to reclaim the personal power that we surrender to the other person when we hold onto resentment. It means refusing to let what happened in the past steal our current and future joy.

Forgiveness does not mean pretending the transgression doesn't matter. It does not require us to resume the relationship. In fact, we do not even need to tell our transgressor that we have forgiven them. Forgiving my abuser does not mean that his behavior was understandable. Even if he had been abused, he could have chosen not to inflict his wounds on me. I didn't bury the memories of what happened; I just stopped carrying the shame attached to them. Decades later, I came face-to-face with my abuser. Freed from my shame, I looked him straight in the face —but he refused to meet my gaze. Just before his eyes flicked away, I saw *his* shame was still active in his field. In that moment, I felt a rush of gratitude for the forgiveness that enabled me to heal.

Some experts stipulate conditions for forgiveness: If the transgression was slight or the damage unintentional, then forgiveness may be an option—but only if the transgressor apologizes first. I disagree, since waiting for an apology puts the power in someone else's hands.

Family members of the people murdered at the Emanuel African Methodist Episcopal Church in South Carolina were both praised and criticized for their swift forgiveness of the shooter. While many people admired their grace, others accused them of disrespecting the memory of their loved ones. But those family members understood that forgiveness had nothing to do with the shooter. Forgiveness meant releasing the energy-blocking emotions that could damage their health.

Our role is not to sit in judgment of others. Even the jury in a criminal trial is not tasked with determining the defendant's guilt or innocence. Their responsibility is to assess whether the prosecutor provided sufficient evidence to substantiate their case beyond a reasonable doubt.

Perhaps someday I might experience something that I cannot forgive—but when I read about families of murder victims forgiving their loved one's killer, it makes me wonder if everything might be forgivable. Certainly, the health benefits make it worth trying.

What does forgiveness mean to you? Do you agree with

Wanda that some things are unforgivable? If so, where do you draw the line?

Is there a wound in your burden bag that forgiveness could heal? Is there an emotional cost to you that comes from withholding your forgiveness?

Consider the mindset of your transgressor. What beliefs, values, and experiences might their behavior reflect? Perhaps, like Lori who lies easily, their experience instilled values that are different from yours.

Is it possible that they did not mean to offend you? Perhaps they didn't understand your mindset, such as when I initially declined tea while visiting my new Middle Eastern friends. Or perhaps they are like my New York colleagues who hurl barbs at one another.

If something in your burden bag feels unforgivable, start by forgiving smaller things. When someone cuts me off in traffic, I remind myself that I have accidentally done the same thing myself. "Perhaps they didn't see me," I think. Or perhaps they are dealing with a stressful situation that makes it hard for them to concentrate on their driving. "I forgive you," I say aloud. Then I forgive myself for getting angry.

Releasing Perfectionism

A quick glance at the clock on the dashboard reminded me how late I was as I headed to a book club meeting. I had not been to the host's house before. Considering that she lived across town, and it was evening rush hour, I'd meant to leave earlier to allow more time. Forty-five minutes later, I was circling through her neighborhood, feeling my anxiety climb. Finally, I pulled over in front of a house that I had passed twice earlier—only this time, the GPS announced that I had arrived. "Strange," I thought, noticing the absence of cars in the driveway. "Everyone else should be here already."

Pulling out my phone to double-check the address, I realized that the book club meeting had been the night before. As I turned my car toward home, I said aloud, "It's OK. I forgive myself for making a mistake." The sensation was like pulling a plug from a tub of water. All the irritation—at the wasted time, wasted gas, poor GPS directions, and embarrassment over missing the meeting drained away. I told myself that running late was a gift, because at least it spared me the added embarrassment of knocking on the host's front door. That's when I noticed that the twilight sky was full of beautiful purples and soft oranges with tiny stars winking awake. I felt grateful that the long drive home allowed me to enjoy the colorful sunset.

Forgiving my abuser opened the door to forgiving myself. At work, I used to scrutinize every deliverable with a fine-tooth comb. Everything my team produced had to be perfect. Before hitting the Send button, I would reread every email multiple times. Slide decks had to be accurate and aesthetically pleasing. The margins had to be even, and the bullets perfectly aligned. A member of my team once told me that we could accomplish more if I wasn't such a perfectionist. Although he considered me nitpicky, I prided myself on my attention to detail. It annoyed me that other people could brush off their mistakes so easily.

Eventually, though, I was forced to acknowledge that my perfectionism was causing me unnecessary stress. I had to ask myself, "What is the mindset behind this pattern of behavior?" I uncovered a limiting belief that mistakes are bad. I recalled how my dad belittled me when I said or did something he didn't like. When I was around five years old, he criticized me for sloppy coloring. Although he rarely interacted with me, Dad took a crayon from me that day and proceeded to show me the "right" way to color.

As you know, we manufacture our mindset, which means that we can also reprogram it. Through affirmations and journaling, I released the belief that mistakes are bad. Although I still experience a momentary cringe when I make a mistake, I immediately remind myself that perfectionism is unrealistic and outdated programming. I say to myself (aloud if possible), "I forgive myself." Boy, that feels amazing!

Research indicates that perfectionism is on the rise, particularly among people between the ages of sixteen and twenty-five, possibly fueled by social media. Fear of making mistakes contributes to chronic stress and can degrade our performance. Recovering from perfectionism raises our vibe and improves our health. Self-acceptance is a prerequisite to authentic and loving relationships.

How readily do you forgive yourself when you make a mistake?

If you struggle with self-forgiveness, try reprogramming your mindset with affirmations such as "I release unrealistic expectations of myself," or "I love and accept myself just as I am." For added effectiveness, look at yourself in the mirror as you recite your affirmations.

You Can't Take It with You

We've all heard the saying "You can't take it with you." The expression really hit home with me after my mom passed away. She had owned an antique store, so her home was tastefully decorated with beautiful high-quality furniture in addition to family heirlooms passed down through generations.

I selected a few things to keep and invited relatives to take whatever they wanted. The rest was donated or sold at auction. Although it meant letting go of some beautiful and sentimental possessions, I didn't want more stuff. Other family members—reluctant to part with Mom's things—filled their garages and basements. They couldn't understand how I could part with her stuff so easily.

Clutter is a vibe crusher. Since learning to see everything as vibrating energy, I view excessive material possessions as an energetic burden. As much as marketing experts try to convince us otherwise, the truth is that our stuff weighs us down. An accumulation of objects can create energetic congestion in the space around us—even lovely items with sentimental value.

I used to work next door to a man who kept reams of printouts stacked floor to ceiling along all the walls in his office and on the surface of his desk. One day, I walked into his office to speak to him and was overcome by queasiness. I didn't stay long, and from then on, I stood in the doorway if I wanted to converse with him. Knowing what I know now, I attribute my discomfort to the oppressive congestion created by all those stacks of paper.

On the other hand, my friend Barb has a clutter-free home that allows energy to flow freely. When I step into her house, I feel so peaceful. I am on a mission to achieve her level of household Zen.

Remember, our thoughts and emotions radiate outward so far that other people can detect them. When we are in an open area, such as outdoors, that electromagnetic energy can freely travel away from us. In a confined space, however, that energy is bouncing off nearby objects, careening around the room, and bouncing back into us. The popularity of minimalism illustrates the energetic relief we experience when our vibes have space to roam.

How would you describe the energy in your living space? Is it expansive or constricted? How does the energy of your living space affect your personal energy? Do you feel light and open or heavy and closed? Do you have stuff that you never use but are holding onto in case you need it someday? If your space would benefit, schedule a day to tackle some serious decluttering. If letting go of items is a challenge, start small by cleaning out a drawer or closet. Notice how it makes you feel energetically. Perhaps you will feel inspired to clear out larger spaces. Avoid moving your stuff to a storage facility; just relocating it isn't the same as releasing it.

I want to emphasize that this advice does not apply to people who suffer from hoarding, which is a serious mental health condition. People who hoard need compassionate professional support to separate from their possessions. If you or someone you know is dealing with a hoarding disorder, consult the National Alliance on Mental Health or similar organization.

While Mom's possessions brought her pleasure when she was alive, she couldn't take them with her when she passed. Wherever our souls go when they leave our human bodies, they have no need for antique china and handcrafted tables. Eventually, I will follow Mom, leaving all my precious things behind; the fewer the better, so my children aren't burdened with them.

And—just like family heirlooms—we can't keep our burden bag forever. While we may have dutifully carried some emotional baggage since childhood, once we come to the end of our days, we must leave it on the platform when we board the train for our journey to the afterlife. Even resentment for apparently unforgivable transgressions is left behind. So, if we have to release our burden bag at some point anyway, why not just do it now?

Using Tapping to Release our Burdens

Psychologist Roger Callahan had been treating "Mary" for aquaphobia, an intense fear of water, for nearly two years, but she was still afraid to go near a filled bathtub. During an exposure therapy session in 1980, Mary became queasy with anxiety. Callahan directed Mary to use her fingertips to tap on the acupuncture point below the center of each eye, which is associated with the stomach meridian, hoping that it would relieve Mary's nausea. To their mutual astonishment, after a few minutes of tapping, Mary suddenly declared her aquaphobia cured. To prove it, she marched outside and stuck her hand in Callahan's swimming pool. When Mary was interviewed thirty years later, her aquaphobia had not returned.

Recall from earlier that the primo vascular system—thread-like vessels that run throughout our body—aligns with the location of the energy meridians. Sprinkled along the meridians are minuscule bundles called *primo nodes*, which match the insertion points used in acupuncture. Acupressure involves stimulating these nodes with our fingertips instead of inserting needles. When Mary tapped beneath her eyes, she was stimulating acupoint number one on the stomach meridian.

After extensive trial-and-error, Callahan concluded that the appropriate acupoints to tap varied depending on his patients' issues. This led Callahan to develop the first tapping protocol, which he named Thought Field Therapy (TFT).[7] Eventually, Callahan settled on eleven meridian points. He created a chart to determine which meridian points to tap and in what sequence. Conditions addressed by TFT include general anxiety, phobias, depression, trauma, addiction, obsession, physical pain, rage, and self-sabotage. The acupoints used in TFT are listed in the table.

During a TFT session, the acupoints are tapped (or percussed) while the client thinks about the emotion they want to clear—just as Mary's fear of water predominated her mind when she tried tapping that day in Callahan's office. Tapping specific acupoints sends a calming signal to the alarm center in the brain, deactivating the fight or flight response. When we think about what bothers us and tap at the same time, it decouples the stress response from the disturbing thought or memory.

Tapping does not erase memories; it just neutralizes the "fight or flight" response. After a tapping session, the client can recall a traumatic event or engage in formerly fearful activities while remaining calm. Anecdotal reports of TFT's effectiveness led to its widespread use across the mental health community, despite the complexity of the algorithm and lack of scientific research at the time.

Thought Field Therapy (TFT)

Tapping Location	Meridian / Acupoint	Imbalance
Beginning point of eyebrow	Bladder 2	Fear, resentment, anger, jealousy, repressed emotions
Outer edge of eyebrow	Gallbladder 1	Anger, frustration, rage
Under eye	Stomach 1	Worry, confusion, low self-esteem
Under nose	Governing 27	Negativity, self-destructive behaviors
Under lip	Conception Vessel 24	Sorrow, shame, unprocessed emotions
Below collarbone	Kidney 27	Fear, ear and dental problems
Side of ribcage four inches below armpit	Spleen 21	Digestive issues, fatigue
Inside of little finger near base of nail bed	Heart 9	Anxiety, loneliness, insomnia
Thumb side of index finger near base of nail bed	Large Intestine 1	Grief, sadness, letting go
Side of hand below base of little finger	Small Intestine 3	Sadness, self-deprecation
Back of hand between base of little finger and ring finger	Triple Warmer 3	Anxiety

Callahan's student, Gary Craig, refined TFT to create the Emotional Freedom Technique (EFT) in 1995. EFT uses the same nine acupoints, regardless of the patient's issues. Craig added a personalized script to help the client focus on the emotion that they want to clear. For example, someone like Mary would say, "This fear of water," while tapping.

Craig documented EFT in a manual consistent with guidelines from the American Psychological Association (APA), which opened the door to formal research studies. So far, over 300 studies have been published in peer-reviewed journals. A majority of studies concluded that EFT was not only effective, but that it also often worked faster and lasted longer than traditional therapies. For more information about EFT research, refer to the book *The Science Behind Tapping* by Peta Stapleton, Ph.D.

The Trauma Tapping Technique

Gunilla Hamne, a Swedish journalist and filmmaker, was interested in using EFT to help the survivors of war, genocide, and natural disasters whom she met in her travels. Unfortunately, she did not know the native language well enough—nor did she have the bandwidth—to develop EFT scripts. She needed a version that was language-independent and simple enough that people could teach it to each other.

In 2007, Hamne partnered with EFT expert Dr. Carl Johnson to develop the Trauma Tapping Technique (TTT). Together, they traveled to Rwanda, where TTT was used with survivors of the genocide that occurred twelve years before. Anyone can use TTT to counteract the symptoms of anxiety. Even children can master the simple steps.

You can use this technique to release any form of energy that is stuck in your field, such as disturbing emotions and repetitive thoughts. If there is an emotion that you could not release using the Burden Bag exercise, try tapping on it.

Follow the steps below or practice along with me using the video in this book's online companion. If tapping a point is uncomfortable, gently massage it until the discomfort eases.

1. Take a moment to notice how you feel. Do you feel your emotions in a particular area of your body—for example tension in your temples or fluttering in your gut?
2. Rate your discomfort on a scale between one and ten, with ten being intensely upset.
3. Begin with a few rounds of Intentional Breathing. Continue to take long, slow breaths while tapping on the meridian points.
4. Tap on each acupoint seven to ten times beginning on the outside edge of one hand (the side opposite the thumb) with the fingertips of the other hand.
5. Proceed through the tapping sequence listed below.
6. After the first round, take two deep diaphragmatic breaths.
7. Repeat the tapping sequence again, beginning with the outside edge of the hand and ending with two deep diaphragmatic breaths.
8. Check in with your emotions and rate your discomfort now by picking a number between one and ten that matches how you feel after tapping. If your discomfort is higher than two, repeat the tapping sequence again.
9. After your final round, you may want to journal about your experience.

Tapping Sequence

A. outside edge of hand
B. inside of both eyebrows
C. on the temple bone at the outside of each eye
D. on the bone under the eyes
E. in the indent under the nose
F. in the indent under the bottom lip
G. both sides of the chest in the divot below the collarbone and above the first rib

H. three inches below the armpit with the palm of the hand
I. inside the little finger next to the base of the nail
J. inside the fourth finger next to the base of the nail
K. inside the middle finger next to the base of the nail
L. inside the index finger next to the base of the nail
M. outside the thumb next to the base of the nail

In 2010, Hamne and Swedish therapist Ulf Sandstrom established The Peaceful Heart Network (PHN), a nonprofit organization headquartered in Sweden. PHN is bringing TTT to communities around the world—from a Syrian refugee camp in Greece, to a prison in Rwanda, orphaned Ukrainian children in Poland, an addiction recovery program in a Virginia jail, wildfire survivors in California, and tornado victims in Nepal. To learn more about TTT, visit the PHN website at peacefulheart.se.

Tapping can be effective even if some points are skipped or tapped in a different sequence. Think of TTT as emotional first aid—a Band-Aid for a minor injury. If we are upset about an argument with a family member, or finances or traffic, or our child is upset about something that happened at school, TTT is an appropriate technique for releasing those emotions. However, just as home care cannot replace the critical intervention necessary to stabilize a serious wound, TTT is not a replacement for professional mental healthcare in situations of severe trauma.

If you are in a situation that is not conducive to a full tapping sequence, just tap on the hand points. It is also effective to firmly but gently squeeze or massage each acupoint for twenty to thirty seconds instead of tapping on it. To build familiarity with TTT, practice every day for seven days. Use the Intentional Release with Tapping Practice Tracker—available in the back of this book or in the online companion—to document your experience.

How to Release Persistent Energetic Blockages

In this chapter, we discovered that clinging to past resentments, regrets, and old wounds can recreate energetic blockages that were previously cleared. Analyzing the contents of our burden bag enables us to release them for good. Forgiveness and TTT are effective techniques for releasing stuck energy. We also learned that releasing excessive material possessions improves the flow of life-force energy in our living space.

Tips to release persistent energetic blockage:

1. Write this chapter's intention (*I intend to release energetic blockages*) on a piece of paper and tape it to your bathroom mirror. Take a moment every morning to decide how you will practice the intention in the day ahead. At the end of the day, congratulate yourself for taking action to cultivate your personal power.
2. Remember that trying to suppress low-vibe emotions keeps them in our biofield where they can lead to physical disease. Instead, focusing attention on your feelings is the fastest way to release them.
3. Use the Burden Bag Release Exercise to unload emotional burdens.
4. Remember that forgiveness is a gift that you give to yourself. Withholding forgiveness until the other person earns it only adds to *your* burden bag. Strengthen your forgiveness muscle by forgiving small transgressions first.
5. Pay attention to physical pain. What is your body trying to tell you?
6. Improve the energetic flow in your living space by clearing out excess material objects.
7. Build familiarity with the TTT by practicing it every day for seven days. Use the Technique Practice Tracker in the back of the book to document your experience.

8. To learn more about the efficacy of tapping, refer to Dr. Stapleton's book or the PHN website.
9. Retake the Chronic Anxiety Self-Assessment. Log your score in the Self-Assessment Tracker to monitor changes in your stress level over time.
10. Teach the Trauma Tapping Technique to others.

NINE
INTENTIONAL NUTRITION

I intend to nourish my body.

IN MY ANXIOUS GO-GO-GO DAYS, my eating habits exacerbated my poor health. I gravitated toward food that could be eaten with one hand while driving or working at my desk. I bought meal replacement bars by the caseload. I could wolf down a bar in a few quick bites, and if that didn't quell my hunger, I would just eat another one. My second choice was fruit-flavored yogurt. I kept a stash in the fridge at work and a spoon in my desk drawer. I would buy fresh fruit occasionally, but the juice would leave a sticky residue on my keyboard. Although I used to teach a class on how to read nutrition labels, I avoided looking at them myself. It made it easier to ignore the fact that the meal bars were laced with unpronounceable chemicals, while a five-ounce carton of the yogurt I chose contained a tablespoon of added sugar.

An expensive car may have a sophisticated engine, but its performance is affected by the quality of the fuel in the tank. So, too, our overall wellness relies on healthful eating.

As I mentioned earlier, when energy healing entered my life, I began to see everything as vibrating energy—including my food. As my mindset shifted, I gravitated toward foods that I perceived as high-frequency. Part of the transition to the new, calm me involved changing the way I was eating. Instead of selecting food based on convenience, I now prioritize nutritional value. Fortunately, I have discovered many foods that are both convenient and nutritious.

In this chapter we will explore the nutritional basics of macronutrients, learn how to make informed food choices, and overcome food cravings. Intentional nutrition is about raising our awareness of how what we eat affects our energetic health.

The Food Frontier

Nutrition can be confusing; often, we are given conflicting advice. For many years, we were assured that moderate alcohol consumption was safe; a glass of red wine with dinner could even be beneficial for heart health! But then in 2025, the U.S. Surgeon General issued an advisory linking alcohol consumption to cancer.

So, how do we know what to believe? It's important to question the trustworthiness of our sources of information. That's why I only consider studies published in peer-reviewed journals. In addition, I check how recently the study was conducted, how many people participated, whether there was a control group (such as in the housekeeper study referenced in Chapter 7) and who paid for the study (usually noted below the conclusion section). A research review (also known as a meta-analysis) compares results across dozens of similar studies, thereby increasing the population size.

The health impact of food is inherently difficult to study. Unlike with rats confined to a lab, researchers have to rely on participants' self-reported eating habits; for example, how much alcohol they admit to consuming. In addition, a participant who was eating poorly before the study will experience more dramatic improvements than someone who was already eating a balanced diet. Conditions such as cardiovascular disease or Type-2 diabetes take decades to develop, and few studies last that long. While they attempt to account for variables such as medical histories, rarely (if ever) do researchers consider the biofield health of participants—which, as we know, can have a significant impact on our well-being.

The Three Macronutrients

We humans tend to sift and sort things into compartments to make them easier to understand. Consider our approach to the human body. We segregate it into a collection of systems: cardiovascular, nervous, endocrine, skeletal and so forth. Yet, our body functions as an integrated whole, blissfully unaware of these textbook categories.

The nutrients in our food are divided into macronutrients and micronutrients according to their chemical composition. Macronutrients are proteins, carbohydrates (carbs), and fats. Micronutrients are vitamins and minerals. Entire books have been dedicated to micronutrients, so I am not going to dive into those here.

There's a tendency to refer to a particular food as a protein or a carb. But—with the notable exception of meat—every food provides all three macronutrients. There are carbs in nuts and protein in bread. It may surprise you that the amount of protein in two slices of wheat bread is comparable to a cup of skim milk. Lean ground beef, on the other hand, provides protein and fat but zero carbs.

There's also a tendency to praise or condemn a macronutrient; for example, protein is good, and carbs are bad. This is a gross misunderstanding, unfortunately. The nutritional quality of a food is much more complicated than its macronutrient content.

Macronutrients

Food	Carbs	Protein	Fat
1/4 cup raw, unsalted almonds	10	11	23
1 cup fat-free or skim dairy milk	12.1	8.4	.2
1 cup raw spinach	3.6	3	0
1 cup cooked lentils	38.6	17.9	.7
1/2 package Nasoya extra firm tofu	2	8	4
1 tablespoon Walmart almond butter	3	3.5	8.5
2 slices whole wheat bread	27.6	7.9	2.3
1/4 pound 90 percent lean ground beef	0	18.2	12.8

Data is from USDA Food Central database
https://fdc.nal.usda.gov/food-search

How Much Protein Do I Need?

According to the Harvard School of Public Health, there are at least 10,000 different types of proteins in the human body. Our body uses protein in many ways, but in the simplest terms, protein serves as the building blocks for making and repairing tissue, bone, blood, and organ cells.

Chemically, proteins are chains of amino acids arranged in various configurations. There are over twenty different types of amino acids. Imagine the pearl necklaces in a jewelry store display case. They may be various lengths, or made of different types of pearls such as saltwater, freshwater, or cultured. Just as the jeweler can combine the pearls from two short necklaces to create a long one, your body can manufacture most of the proteins it needs by reconfiguring the amino acids from your last meal.

There are nine amino acids, however, that the body cannot manufacture—we can only get these essential amino acids from our diet: histidine, isoleucine, leucine, lysine, methionine, phenylalanine, threonine, tryptophan, and valine. If a particular food provides all nine of the essential amino acids, it is considered a complete protein. Although the easiest way to ensure that you are consuming adequate amounts of essential amino acids is to eat a variety of foods, rest assured that plant foods are complete proteins.

In the Standard American Diet (SAD), protein takes center stage at every meal. As a result, many Americans eat more than the recommended amount of protein. To calculate your recommended amount, multiply your weight in pounds by 0.36 or use the free USDA calculator available online. I weigh 133 pounds, so my recommended daily allowance (RDA) for protein is 48 grams. Protein requirements are higher for athletes, seniors, and pregnant and lactating women. Too much of a good thing can be detrimental to your health, however, as excessive dietary protein is linked to kidney stones, osteoporosis, heart disease and cancer.[1]

All protein is not created equal. The source of the protein you consume is just as—if not more—important than the quantity. As a health coach, I frequently encounter the misperception that we need to eat meat to ensure an adequate intake of protein. While it's true that, ounce for ounce, meat provides more protein than plant-based sources, animal proteins (including cheeses) are high in saturated fat. On the other hand, plant-based proteins such as beans, legumes, nuts, and seeds are low in saturated fat and provide the added benefit of fiber, which is absent from animal protein.

Another concern regarding animal-based proteins is the unreported substances that may be present. Cows, pigs, and chickens are fed hormone-laced grain to shorten time to market. Dairy cows are given hormones to increase milk production. Due to crowded living conditions, livestock are often treated with antibiotics to limit the spread of diseases.

I switched to plant-based protein over fifteen years ago. For example, I typically break my overnight fast with a homemade concoction of rolled oats, chia seeds, and ground flaxseeds soaked in homemade almond and hemp seed milk, and topped with fresh fruit. A serving has 26 grams of protein (54 percent of my recommended amount of protein in one meal) plus 21(of the recommended 28) grams of fiber. Refer to the online companion to this book for recipes including overnight oats.

Should I Avoid Carbs?

The term *carbohydrate* was introduced by the Commission on the Nomenclature of Organic Chemistry in 1969. Chemically, carbs are composed of carbon, oxygen and hydrogen molecules in various configurations. Fiber, starch and all types of sugar fall under the umbrella of carbs.

Fiber, the indigestible part of plants, is an essential component of a well-rounded diet. Our intestine is home to trillions of microorganisms—bacteria, viruses, fungi, and microbes—that form our gut microbiome. Some of these microbes are probiotics, which play a critical role in digesting food, producing essential nutrients, and regulating immune function as well as cholesterol and glucose levels. High-fiber foods are prebiotics, which nourish the healthful probiotic bacteria in our gut. Without fiber to ferment, probiotics will die, allowing unhealthy pathogens to flourish. An imbalance in gut bacteria, known as *dysbiosis*, can lead to neurological issues, abdominal pain, and weight gain. Emerging research strongly indicates a link between dysbiosis and mental health conditions such as depression, as well as autoimmune diseases such as rheumatoid arthritis.[2,3]

Fiber supports smooth functioning of the digestive system and provides a sense of fullness that helps us avoid overeating. It reduces the risk of excess body fat, colon cancer, Type 2 diabetes, and cardiovascular disease. Most Americans consume about 15 grams of fiber a day, which is below the recommended daily amount of 25–30 grams. If your diet is high in animal protein (meat, eggs, and dairy), you may not be getting enough fiber. Ensuring that you are consuming an adequate amount of fiber every day is critical for intentional nutrition.

Introduce fiber into your diet gradually to allow your digestive system to adjust. If your gut microbiome is unbalanced, your body needs time to restore the colonies of probiotics that feed on fiber.

There are other types of sugar in carbs besides the white stuff you stir into your coffee. Just as proteins are chains of amino acids, sugars are chains of saccharides. Our digestive system converts the sugars we eat into glucose. We need glucose to survive, as it is the fuel that energizes our brain, nervous system, and red blood cells. Carbs are the body's preferred energy source, but if we restrict our carbohydrate intake, our body will survive by manufacturing glucose from protein and fat although the process can be stressful for the kidneys.

Without getting into all the different forms of sugar, the important thing to remember is that simple sugars are short chains of one or two saccharides, while complex sugars are longer chains of three or more saccharides. The table sugar you stir into coffee is a disaccharide—a form of simple sugar made by combining two monosaccharides together.

Glucose is also a simple sugar composed of one saccharide (a monosaccharide). Because they are chemically similar, simple sugars like table sugar convert to glucose quickly during digestion. On the other hand, it takes our body longer to convert long chains of complex sugars into glucose.

The presence of fiber slows the glucose conversion process even more. Eat an apple and glucose will dribble into your bloodstream as the fiber in the apple slows digestion. A steady stream of glucose staves off hunger. Drink a cup of apple juice, which has the sugar equivalent of three apples but no fiber, and your glucose level will spike before crashing.

A glucose spike is a rapid infusion of glucose that exceeds what the body needs to feed hungry cells. The excess glucose is stored as fat, leading to a severe drop in glucose levels and the urge to eat again. Years of frequent glucose spikes increase the risk for Type 2 diabetes.

I'm not recommending that you eliminate all forms of simple sugar from your diet; that may not be a realistic goal. I encourage you, however, to limit your consumption of simple sugars, which promote the growth of proteobacteria—a gut microbe associated with inflammation. As a former sugar fiend, in my experience, it is possible to wean ourselves off sweet treats over time. If you occasionally indulge in food high in simple sugars, you can flatten the glucose spike by eating a fibrous food first.

Not all carbs are created equal. From an organic chemistry perspective, broccoli is primarily carbs—but so is a donut. When we consider nutritional value, broccoli provides micronutrients such as vitamin C, vitamin A, beta carotene, and fiber, while the donut lacks micronutrients and—loaded with simple sugar—spikes blood glucose, contributing to body fat.

On the shelves in the center of the grocery store, we find boxes of highly processed, carb-laden, low-fiber foods such as crackers, breakfast cereals, breads, and snack items. These products have much of the fiber removed to extend shelf life. Many are high in simple sugar to improve palatability, which keeps consumers coming back for more. These are the foods that give carbs a bad name. Make it a habit to check the fiber content and amount of added sugar on nutritional labels.

The Skinny on Fat

Just as with the other macronutrients, dietary fat plays an important role in nourishing our body. The fat we eat builds cell membranes, produces hormones, and absorbs fat-soluble vitamins. It also generates energy.

As with protein and carbs, there are different kinds of fat. Fats—or fatty acids—are primarily chains of carbon and hydrogen molecules in various configurations. If all the hydrogen receptors on a carbon molecule are occupied, the fat is saturated. Saturated fats are solid at room temperature. Examples include lard, coconut oil, the strip of fat along the edge of a steak, or the yellowish globs on raw chicken. Fried and fast foods, processed meat products like sausage, some nuts (cashews, macadamia, and Brazil), dairy products like cheese and ice cream, as well as processed bakery products tend to be high in saturated fat.

In unsaturated fats, some of the hydrogen receptors are unoccupied. If one receptor is empty, the fat is monounsaturated. If more than one receptor is available, though, then the fat is polyunsaturated. Unsaturated fats are liquid at room temperature. Plant-based oils such as olive, canola, sunflower, corn, soybean, and flaxseed oils are unsaturated. Food sources of unsaturated fats include nuts (almonds, hazelnuts, pecans, and walnuts), seeds (pumpkin, flax, and sesame), and avocados.

As with essential amino acids, there are two types of unsaturated fats that our body cannot manufacture. We can only get these essential fatty acids from our diet. One is alpha-linolenic acid (a type of omega-3 fatty acid), while the other is linoleic acid (a type of omega-6 fatty acid).

More research is needed, but omega-3s appear to reduce the risk of cardiovascular disease and some forms of cancer. Walnuts, some legumes, hemp seed, flaxseed, chia seeds, deep-sea fish, and leafy greens are sources of omega-3s. Foods rich in omega-6 fatty acids include sunflower seeds, pumpkin seeds, almonds, pecans, pistachios, and legumes.

Omega-6s are also found in plant-based cooking oils (safflower oil, sunflower oil, corn oil, and soybean oil) which are often used in processed foods. So, while intentional effort is needed to ensure adequate intake of omega-3s, most people consume more than enough omega-6s.

It is generally accepted that diets high in fats—especially saturated fats—contribute to cardiovascular issues. Yet, some studies indicate that people may benefit from a diet high in saturated fat. As mentioned earlier, nutrition is a tricky topic to research. Although someday researchers may discover that saturated fat is safe to consume, I recommend choosing sources of unsaturated fat until more is known.

Compared to the other macronutrients, we need a smaller quantity of fat because it is energy-dense, with nine calories per gram compared to four calories per gram for protein and carbs. Researchers have observed that rats fed a low-fat diet will eat more food to compensate for the caloric deficit. Unlike the other macronutrients, the recommended daily amount is a percentage of overall caloric intake. The Acceptable Macronutrient Distribution Range (AMDR) for fat is 30–40 percent of total energy intake for children aged 1–3 years, 25–35 percent for children aged 4–18 years, and 20–35 percent for adults.

Make it a habit to compare the amount of saturated and unsaturated fat on nutritional labels. Choose foods low in saturated fat. Cook with oils that are liquid at room temperature. I rely on seeds—hemp, flax, and chia—to add essential omega-3 fatty acids to my diet. My breakfast concoction includes all three. Combining these seeds with fresh dates makes delicious energy bars. Chia seeds may be combined with water to make a gel-like egg substitute for baking. Hemp seeds increase the creaminess of smoothies. Refer to this book's online companion for recipe ideas.

The Daily Food Diary Exercise

Logging your food consumption for a day is a great way to ensure that you are consuming adequate amounts of fiber and macronutrients. It can be a time-consuming practice—so while it may be enlightening, it is not necessary to do it every day.

There's a worksheet in the back of this book and in the online companion that you can use to track your nutritional intake for a day and compare it to the recommended amounts for your age, gender, and activity level.

As you focus on your dietary intake, consider how your mindset may influence your food choices. What foods did you eat growing up? Do certain foods or aromas trigger pleasant memories? Could your emotions be influencing your preferences for particular foods?

The Energy of Food

As you know, everything is energy. Fresh produce is from a living plant, so it makes sense that our food would have the highest vibration in its natural state.

I fill my cart with fresh produce when I go grocery shopping. As soon as I get home, I wash my produce before storing it in containers designed to extend freshness. There are always bowls of washed produce in my fridge. This saves me time when preparing meals and reduces food waste.

Preparation matters. From a nutritional perspective, there's a big difference between eating broccoli raw, roasted, steamed, or boiled to a mush and drowned in butter. Depending on how it is prepared, produce is low in added sugar and saturated fat and high in fiber. Eating produce raw is the best option—but lightly cooked with minimal added fat and salt is okay, especially when making the transition. I make the effort to consume fresh produce at every meal.

The more a food is processed, the less life-force energy it radiates. Canning, freezing, and cooking reduce the vibration to an extent that I find acceptable in moderation. I keep frozen veggies on hand for emergencies.

Food that has been highly processed—pulverized into flour

and mixed with chemicals that are only available in commercial production facilities—feels energetically dead to me. Because commercial processing removes so many of the micronutrients, the vitamins listed on the label are added back in prior to packaging. Those meal bars and fruity yogurt cups that I used to eat every day are no longer on the menu for me.

Starting with your next meal, consider the energetic radiance of the food you are eating. How alive is it? Pay attention to how your food affects your vibe.

Look for ways to add more fresh produce into your diet. Buy only as much as you can consume in the next week or less. Clean it straight away and employ strategies to extend the shelf life. Soft-skinned fruits like berries get a thorough rinse in cold water. I remove grapes from the vine first so to expose more of the surface area. Fruits with a peel such as apples and oranges soak for several minutes in a bath of cold water and baking soda (1 teaspoon baking soda per 2 cups water) before a thorough rinse. After destemming, leafy greens like kale also get a soaking and rinse before a turn in the salad spinner to remove excess moisture. Hard vegetables like potatoes get scrubbed with a vegetable brush. I don't wash mushrooms until I am ready to use them. Prewashed lettuces and micro greens go straight into the fridge.

For storage, I use containers designed to keep produce fresh. Potatoes and onions are stored in a dark closet, although not on the same shelf as they can accelerate each other's aging. Not only does it save time preparing meals, but I'm more likely to use produce that is clean and ready to eat.

The Daily Produce Exercise

When you feel ready to add more fiber to your diet, challenge yourself to eat at least five servings of produce every day for seven days. Raw or lightly cooked are okay. Experiment with different types of produce. I base my choices on what looks freshest, is in season, or on sale. Eating a variety of produce is crucial. Aim to consume thirty different types of plants every week. There's a worksheet in the back of the book and in the online companion that you can use to track your produce intake and take notes on your experience.

How to Evaluate Processed Foods

By law, processed foods display standard nutrition facts on the label. A trip to the store is not necessary for comparison shopping. The nutrition facts for most—if not all—branded products are available online. When evaluating a product, I focus on a few key items.

First, look at the saturated fat content. The ideal amount will vary depending on the product, but our goal is to avoid saturated fat. Below that is the amount of trans fat. If it is anything other than zero, do not buy the product.

Next, check the amount of added sugar. We can safely assume this represents simple sugar that was added to the product to enhance the taste. Try to find a comparable product that does not contain added sugar. Feel free to ignore total sugars, as complex sugars digest slowly, preventing a glucose spike.

Micronutrients are shown near the bottom. Vitamin D, calcium, iron and potassium are always shown. If a product is high in other particular micronutrients, the manufacturer may choose to list them as well. Honestly, I ignore this section unless I am comparing brands.

Finally, if everything else looks good, check the serving size. If the label indicates that the product contains 12 grams of added sugar, but the serving size is half the amount you typically consume, you are eating 24 grams of sugar.

To check the nutrition content of unprocessed foods, I rely on the USDA's Food Central databases. Many restaurant franchises provide nutrition data for their menu items. If you frequent a particular chain, you may want to look up your favorite dishes.

The Healthy Eating Plate

The Healthy Eating Plate developed by the Harvard T. H. Chan School of Public Health is a straightforward method to ensure a balanced diet.[4] This approach provides a simple ratio that is easy to remember. It is much easier than keeping a food diary.

According to the Healthy Eating Plate, aim for half of what is on your plate at each meal to be vegetables and fruits, one quarter whole grains, and the other quarter healthy protein. Drink plenty of water and limit your intake of sugary drinks.

In addition, Harvard recommends consuming two or fewer servings of dairy a day because it appears to be linked to prostate cancer. Claims regarding bone health are unsubstantiated by scientific research. Plus, the health effects of long-term exposure to the hormones in dairy are uncertain. Compare the labels and you will discover that fortified plant-based milks are higher in calcium than cow's milk.

Note that potatoes are not counted as a vegetable in this plan; because they are high in simple sugar and low in fiber, potatoes trigger a glucose spike. To learn more about the Healthy Eating Plate, visit Harvard's website.

Whole Grains and Lean Proteins

Trying new foods can be intimidating. I get it! It's easier to revert to the same old standbys in the kitchen, especially when time is at a premium. Recall that our survival instinct resists change. But considering that these foods are inexpensive, simple to prepare, and nutritious, that's a healthy return on the time you invest in learning how to prepare them.

I am a big fan of Buddha bowls for a speedy dinner. Simply prepare a whole grain and a lean protein. Add it to a bowl of raw or lightly cooked veggies and top with a homemade dressing made with tahini, miso, or hemp seeds.

Interestingly, many whole grains are surprisingly high in lean protein. In whole grain foods, all three parts of the kernel—the bran, germ, and endosperm—are intact, preserving the nutritional quality and fiber. Whole grains provide *polyphenols*—plant-based compounds associated with reducing inflammation and cholesterol—as well as risks for heart disease, Type 2 diabetes, blood clots, and cancer. Be wary of the "whole grain" claim on food labels (especially for breads and crackers); the food may be made primarily from low-fiber flour and have only a few whole grains sprinkled on top.

My go-to whole grains are oats, quinoa, bulgur, farro, brown rice (white rice is not a whole grain), and barley. Whole grains are easy to prepare by boiling in water on the stovetop for several minutes. If there are multiple brands to choose from, compare the labels; the nutrition content may vary depending on where the plants were grown.

Quinoa was once hailed as sacred by the Incas for its remarkable medicinal properties. It is 15 percent protein and contains all nine essential amino acids. Micronutrients include B vitamins like B2, B6, and B9, as well as essential minerals such as magnesium (which aids in blood sugar regulation and immune system function) and potassium (which supports a healthy heart). Quinoa boasts antioxidant, anti-inflammatory, anti-diabetic, and even anti-cancer properties, thanks to its abundance of *proanthocyanidins*. The phytosterols in quinoa help to reduce cholesterol levels.

When I first started fixing quinoa, I made the mistake of treating it like rice. Believe me, a heaping serving of plain quinoa is decidedly unappetizing! Instead, I will toss it into a bowl of roasted veggies or—my favorite—make a salad with massaged kale, fresh fruit, and a light vinaigrette. Toasted quinoa adds a crunchy topping to salads or soups. You can also add it to homemade granola.

I eat oats several times a week. Oats provide six grams of protein per ½-cup serving. Prepared with milk, the protein amount would be even higher. Also high in antioxidants, micronutrients in oats include manganese, phosphorus, magnesium, copper, iron, zinc, folate and B vitamins—primarily B1 and B5. Many studies have concluded that eating oats reduces cholesterol. If you are short on time in the morning, overnight oats are super easy to mix up the night before and grab on your way out the door.

With five grams of protein in each ¼-cup serving, farro is higher in protein than other whole grains. It is also higher in fiber, so you may want to work your way up to it if you are new to fiber. Farro has been used in weight loss studies because its high fiber content makes it especially filling, and people who eat it tend to consume less food overall.

In addition to whole grains, my favorite sources of lean protein are tofu, tempeh, beans, lentils, and jackfruit. Tofu and tempeh are inexpensive sources of lean protein made from soybeans. Tofu is made by cooking dried soybeans that have been soaked in water and ground to a pulp. After a coagulant made from magnesium or calcium salts is added, the tofu is exposed to high temperatures to pasteurize it. Tempeh is a fermented soy product made by soaking, hulling, boiling, and drying soybeans before adding a bacterial starter. As the beans ferment, they meld together to form a block. Different production methods yield different results, so experiment with brands to find the one you like best.

Since tofu and tempeh are both made from soybeans, they provide similar health benefits. Both provide all nine of the essential amino acids. The vitamins and minerals in tofu include B vitamins (B1, B2, B3, B5, B6 and B12), choline, iron, potassium, zinc, magnesium, phosphorus, copper, selenium, manganese and calcium. In addition to providing 10 percent of the RDA for iron, tempeh is an excellent source of calcium, phosphorus, and manganese.

The American Cancer Society recommends soy products because studies associate soy with lower incidents or recurrences of breast, lung, and prostate cancer.[5] The American Heart Association also recommends soy as long as it is prepared without excess salt, sugar, or saturated fat.[6]

A 2023 review in the journal *Nutrients* encourages athletes to consume tempeh to boost athletic performance and recovery.[7] Six of the amino acids in tempeh promote muscle growth, while another amino acid, L-arginine, limits fat storage. In addition, the microbes in tempeh have been shown to increase muscle mass in the elderly, promote recovery from fatigue, and reduce anxiety.

Both tofu and tempeh are quick and easy to prepare. Tofu is available in different textures or consistencies. Someone once told me that they hated tofu because it was slimy. That sounds to me like they chose the wrong texture for the preparation method; for example, the creamy consistency of silken tofu is better suited for smoothies and sauces than for a stir fry.

My friend Eliza recalls making fried jackfruit and banana spring rolls with brown sugar in her native Philippines. Native to southeast Asia, jackfruit is the largest tree fruit in the world. Knobby and yellowish-green on the outside, most jackfruit weigh in at 10–25 pounds—although it can grow up to 100 pounds!

The treats that Eliza enjoyed were made from sweet, ripe jackfruit, which is available in the freezer section of grocery stores. But I use unripe jackfruit canned in brine. Its stringy texture shreds like pork, making it a popular meat alternative. Just give it a good rinse in the colander, flake with your fingers, and it is ready for cooking. Sautéed with cumin, chili powder, paprika, onion, bell pepper, and mushrooms, jackfruit makes delicious carnitas. If you find jackfruit products that are precooked and seasoned, be sure to check the label for sodium and added sugar.

From a protein perspective, jackfruit provides six of the nine essential amino acids, as well as arginine and cystine. While most of the calories come from simple sugars, half a cup of unripe jackfruit provides 25 percent of the recommended daily allowance for fiber, thereby avoiding the glucose spike typically associated with sweet treats. Jackfruit is rich in vitamin C and B-complex vitamins, magnesium, potassium, copper, and iron.

According to a 2019 article in the *International Journal of Food Science*, the compounds in jackfruit prevent the formation of cancer cells, stomach ulcers and high blood pressure.[8] Jackfruit also supports eyes, bones, muscles, and nerve functions.

The next time you visit the grocery store, pick up whole grain and lean protein products to try! You can find recipes in this book's online companion.

Why Stress Triggers Cravings

Stress and nutrition have an interdependent relationship. By redirecting our energy to maintaining a state of high alert, chronic stress interferes with our body's ability to extract nutrients from the foods we eat. Some of the nutrients pass through our system undigested. Because the body is not being adequately fueled, our brain stimulates us to eat more food.

With the fuel gauge approaching empty, the body craves simple sugars because they are more readily converted to glucose. The brain creates an irresistible urge for foods like candy, pastries, or potato chips, which flood our bloodstream with glucose. But since our body can only burn so much glucose at a time, the excess is stored as fat. Soon, the amount of glucose in our system dips again and the cycle repeats.

When we are chronically stressed, we tend to reach for ultra-processed foods—foods low in fiber and laced with unpronounceable chemicals. As we discovered earlier, the healthy bacteria in our gut rely on fiber from fresh produce to survive. As healthy bacteria die off, unhealthy bacteria reproduce unchecked. The health impact of the chemicals in ultra-processed food is unknown. Many experts are alarmed by potential dangers, while food manufacturers are demanding more evidence that concern is warranted because their livelihoods are at stake.

It's no secret that what we eat affects how we feel. If we are consuming foods that don't nourish our body, we become lethargic and more vulnerable to stress. So, while stress can lead us on a downward spiral of unhealthy eating, improving our nutrition helps us build resilience to stress.

Improving our eating habits can be tough. Many studies have shown that sugar and highly-processed foods might be as addictive as cocaine. Be gentle with yourself on your journey of intentional eating. By regularly practicing the techniques in this book, you can lower your anxiety baseline. Filling up on nutritious foods may help offset cravings for ultra-processed foods. Avoid bringing ultra-processed foods into your home or workspace.

Tapping has been shown to be effective at combating addictions, from nicotine to food cravings. In a 2017 study out of Australia led by Dr. Stapleton, obese participants were shown photos of tempting foods like pizza, ice cream, and other treats while their brains were scanned using a functional MRI (fMRI).[9] The scans showed significant activity in the area of the brain associated with reward. After eight tapping sessions using EFT over a period of four weeks, participants reported a significant decrease in cravings for what had once been irresistible foods. When the scans were repeated, their neurological response to the photos barely registered—if at all. Follow-up interviews and brain scans a year later confirmed that the participants' food cravings had not returned.

My personal downfall is fatty, salty foods—especially potato chips. I used to buy a family size bag every week. Sometimes, the craving was so strong that I would eat nearly the entire bag in one sitting. Only when my tummy started to hurt could I stop shoving chips in my mouth. Tapping on my chip craving was remarkably effective. Although my husband still buys potato chips, they don't hold the same appeal for me that they used to.

Is there a food that you find particularly enticing? Perhaps—

like me with potato chips—you struggle to resist it? With a few modifications, we can use the Trauma Tapping Technique that we learned in the last chapter to neutralize cravings. In the first step, rate the intensity of your craving on a scale between one and ten, with ten being so intense that it's hard to think of anything else. After completing two rounds of tapping, reevaluate your craving. Repeat the steps until you rate your craving intensity at two or less. Then redirect your flashlight of focus toward your reasons for improving your health. It may help to revisit the whys you wrote down during the Readiness Assessment at the beginning of this book.

Sometimes, food cravings are our body's way of distracting us from painful emotions. If your craving keeps coming back, use your journal to track what situations tend to precede the desire for a particular food.

How to Nourish Your Body

In this chapter, you learned about the three macronutrients: protein, carbs, and fat. We explored the numerous health benefits of fiber, including nourishing our gut microbiome and flattening glucose spikes. We learned that vegetables, fruits, whole grains, and lean proteins have a higher life force energy than ultra-processed products. Stress makes us desire foods high in simple sugars, but we can use tapping to overcome cravings. Tips for nourishing your body:

1. Write this chapter's intention (*I intend to nourish my body*) on a piece of paper and tape it to your bathroom mirror. Take a moment every morning to decide how you will practice the intention in the day ahead. At the end of the day, congratulate yourself for taking action to cultivate your personal power.

2. Use the USDA online calculator to determine your recommended intake of nutrients.
3. Track what you eat in a day using the Food Diary worksheet to compare your actual consumption to the recommended amounts.
4. Once your body has adjusted to eating fiber, challenge yourself to eat at least five servings of produce every day for seven days. Use the Daily Produce Tracker worksheet to track your progress.
5. Use Harvard's Healthy Eating Plate to ensure a balanced intake of vegetables, fruits, whole grains, and lean proteins.
6. Experiment with plant-based sources of protein, which are also high in fiber. If you are new to a high-fiber diet, increase the amounts gradually to allow your digestive system time to adjust.
7. Continue to practice techniques like Intentional Breathing and Grounding to reduce stress that can trigger the desire for foods high in simple sugars.
8. Try tapping to overcome cravings.
9. Refer to the online companion for healthy recipes.
10. Subscribe to my newsletter for the latest findings in nutrition research.
11. Retake the Chronic Anxiety Self-Assessment. Log your score in the Self-Assessment Tracker to monitor changes in your stress level over time.

TEN
INTENTIONAL MOVEMENT

I intend to move my body every day.

IN MY TWENTIES, I loved going to aerobic dance classes. But as work and parenting demanded more of my attention, it became increasingly difficult to change into workout clothes and get to the gym. I didn't have time to work out there and then shower and do my make-up before work, so I would try to go to aerobics class afterward—meaning that I arrived home sweaty and longing for a shower when the rest of the family was ready for dinner. As my responsibilities increased, I found it harder and harder to leave the office in time to make it to the gym. Eventually, I stopped trying.

Sitting at a desk all day took a toll on my physical health. I lost muscle strength and stamina. I felt unsteady carrying the vacuum up and down the stairs. The day I had to ask my son to help me, I knew I needed to improve my physical fitness.

Intentional movement means finding ways to incorporate movement into our daily routine.

The Importance of Movement

It should come as no surprise that movement is important to our wellness. Humans were never meant to sit at desks for hours every day. As busy as we are, we need to be intentional about physical activity. Fortunately, this is easier than some might expect. It is not necessary to visit the gym for hours at a time. And—as we learned from the study with the hotel housekeepers—the movement required to perform household chores and yard work is as effective as structured exercise with the right mindset.

Movement helps our body return to homeostasis after a stressful event. When our nervous system triggers the "fight or flight" alarm, a host of chemicals are released into the bloodstream, including insulin, cortisol, and adrenaline. The activity of running away from—or fighting off—a hungry predator dissipates those chemicals. If you've ever observed a wild animal escape a predatory attack, you may have noticed the animal shaking afterward. This movement helps them reset their nervous system by releasing any residual stress chemicals.

While it may not be appropriate to run away from a disgruntled client, intentional physical activity will have the same beneficial effect. Otherwise, we may still have remnants of "fight or flight" chemicals circulating in our system when the next stressor releases another infusion. Since adrenaline is designed to get us fighting or flighting, an excess amount makes it difficult to relax enough to fall asleep. In the long term these chemicals contribute to fatigue, irritability, digestive issues, cravings, body aches, and memory problems.

Stress chemicals also interfere with our body's absorption of vitamin C, zinc, B vitamins, and magnesium—so even if you are choosing healthy foods or taking a supplement, your body may not be able to utilize the nutrients. Eventually, we are too tired to get off the couch when that is exactly what our body needs the most.

There's a reciprocal relationship between Intentional Movement and other intentions. Our body needs Intentional Nutrition to have the energy to exercise; as movement strengthens our body, we are naturally drawn to healthy foods.

Moderate exercise, dancing, singing, and laughing release "feel-good" chemicals such as endorphins, serotonin, and dopamine, which can have a positive effect on our mental health. These "feel-good" hormones have an opioid-like effect on our brain, elevating our vibe while decreasing pain.

Clinical trials have demonstrated that movement reduces levels of cortisol in the bloodstream, relieving symptoms of anxiety and depression. As our strength and stamina increase, we feel more self-confident about our physical ability, which enhances our self-identity and mindset. Intentional Movement redirects our focus on the physical activity, quieting the chatter of our inner monologue.

Movement flushes toxins from our body and supports our immune system defenses. Lymph is a clear fluid that travels throughout our body via a system of vessels as extensive as the circulatory system. One role of the lymphatic system is garbage collector. Lymph carries away the byproducts of cellular metabolism. Unlike blood—which is pumped throughout the body by the heart—lymph relies on physical activity for circulation. The pressure of our muscles expanding and contracting push lymph fluid through the vessels. Imagine how the garbage would pile up if the trash collectors stopped working.

Along its route, lymph fluid travels through lymph nodes where it is inspected for pathogens like bacteria or viruses, so the immune system can launch an attack against foreign invaders. If the flow of lymph is sluggish due to physical inactivity, pathogens have more time to replicate before our immune system knows they are there.

According to Harvard Medical School, movement improves our cardiovascular health by strengthening the contractions of our heart, increasing the flexibility of our arteries, and moderating our cholesterol.[1] It reduces symptoms of depression and cognitive decline as well as staving off glucose spikes that can lead to Type 2 diabetes.

A 2017 study reported in the journal *Oxidative Medicine and Cellular Longevity* found strong evidence that exercise increases the quality and quantity of healthful bacteria in our gut.[2] This could lead to proliferation of microflora that reduce obesity, metabolic disorders, gastrointestinal disorders, and the risk of colon cancer.

Before starting any exercise program, it is important to check with your doctor first. Never rely on exercise as a replacement for seeing your doctor about specific health concerns. Always listen to your body and go at your own pace. If we jump into a new activity with too much enthusiasm, we risk injuring ourselves. Strive for a duration and frequency that is sustainable for years to come. Stop immediately if you experience pain or dizziness.

The Blowout Technique

This sixty-second technique gets the blood moving and helps to clear stress chemicals from our bloodstream. Follow the steps below or practice along with me using the video in the online companion.

If you feel dizzy, sit down immediately.

1. Begin by standing with your feet parallel and knees slightly bent. Make sure that you have space to swing your arms to the front and to the sides without hitting anything.
2. Inhale sharply through your nose while swinging both arms forward and up to shoulder height.
3. Inhale sharply through your nose again while swinging both arms out to the sides and up to shoulder height.

4. Inhale sharply through your nose a third time while swinging both arms up above your head.
5. Now, exhale all the air sharply through your mouth while folding forward allowing your arms to swing down towards the floor.
6. Repeat steps 2–5 nine more times. Try to move at a pace that will enable you to complete ten rounds in about sixty seconds.
7. On the last round, remain folded forward for a few seconds before placing your hands above your knees and slowly returning to an upright position.

Barriers to Movement

Lack of time is the most frequently cited reason for not exercising. Many of us believe that exercise involves changing into workout clothes, going to the gym for hours, and coming home sweaty. That is how I used to exercise in my twenties. But, again, as we learned from the study with hotel housekeepers, all movement counts toward our fitness level. Start by identifying a five- to ten-minute space in your existing routine for intentional movement. I use the time right before I get dressed for the day to practice yoga in my pajamas.

Accessibility is another barrier. We may not live near a gym, have disposable income to pay for a membership, or live in an area with sidewalks conducive to walking. The weather may be a perceived barrier if it is often too hot or snowy to exercise outdoors. If we have access to the internet or a DVD player, though, you can exercise in the comfort of your home when it is convenient for your schedule. With so many free instructor-led practices available online, you should be able to find some certified instructors you like.

Our mindset can interfere with our commitment to intentional movement. Many of my clients accept physical deterioration as natural. Perhaps this mindset sprang from the experience of observing their parents and grandparents grow old. They resign themselves to painful joints and limited mobility. He is no longer with us, but whenever I would ask my friend David how he was doing, his standard reply was, "It's terrible getting older." But a long, slow decline into frailty is optional. No matter how old or out of shape we are, we can improve our fitness level. As shaman Alberto Villoldo states, "Growing older is inevitable. Aging is preventable." What is your mindset regarding physical activity? How has your past experience shaped your attitude toward exercise?

When we introduce intentional movement into our life, we may feel a powerful urge to stop. Remember, our survival instinct is to naturally resist change.

Mental rehearsal is widely used by professional athletes to enhance competitive performance. Golfer Jack Nicklaus and boxer Mohammad Ali both credit visualization for their success. In an experiment with Olympic skiers, researchers found that the appropriate muscles were firing as the skier imagined themselves navigating a specific slope. A controlled randomized study of nursing students conducted in 2021 found that mentally rehearsing cardiopulmonary resuscitation (CPR) shortened reaction times and reduced errors compared to students in the control group. Use the Focuser Technique and mental rehearsal to ease the transition to a more active you.

If you feel pain at all during exercise, stop immediately to avoid injury. Choose a different form of movement or make adjustments. For example, although I practice intermediate-level yoga every day, I adjust the poses to avoid aggravating my cranky left knee. We want to push through mental resistance but take pain seriously.

As we touched on at the beginning of this book, any transformational change requires understanding our *readiness* for change. What are your *whys* and *why nots* for moving every day? What sacrifices are required to make space in your busy life for physical activities? You may want to revisit the Readiness

Assessment from the perspective of Intentional Movement. Remember that we all have twenty-four hours in a day. It's not a matter of how much time we have as much as it's a matter of how we use that time.

Movements to Try

As you seek to add intentional movement to your day, you may want to experiment with the movement practices listed below. These forms of exercise are great for beginners but also offer continuous challenge as you build stamina and master the simpler forms. All are low-impact, making them joint-friendly. Best of all, they are equally accessible to kids and seniors. Chair classes—where the movements are performed seated—are available for both yoga and qigong.

Yoga

Scholars believe that humans have been practicing yoga since at least 500 BC. Initially, yoga was a spiritual practice originating in India designed to raise awareness of the connection between the individual and universal consciousness. The poses, or *asanas*, that most people associate with yoga were only one aspect of this ancient practice. Although contemporary yoga is widely viewed as exercise, many teachers still include the spiritual aspects. As one of my yoga instructors says, "Yoga is not a workout. Yoga is a work *in*."

There are several different types of yoga. All forms link movement to breath; in other words, a movement starts with an inhale before flowing to the next position on an exhale. Some poses require balancing on one leg, which helps build muscle strength and stability. Hatha yoga is perhaps the most commonly offered style, but class formats may vary by teacher under this umbrella term. Typically, Hatha yoga is considered a good format for beginners, as poses are held for several breaths while the teacher offers guidance on proper alignments. In Ashtanga yoga, the movements tend to keep flowing, making class a little more athletic. Students are expected to know alignment. Yin yoga focuses on stretches, which are held for several minutes, allowing the body to ease into the full expression of the pose.

No special equipment is required to start, although in time you may want a yoga mat, blocks, and a strap. It is best to place your mat on a hard floor, although I practiced on my bedroom rug in the beginning.

If you are new to yoga, look for a beginner-level class that describes proper alignment and breathing. It's important to find someone who encourages you to go at your own pace and rest as needed, and demonstrates options based on your body's structure and mobility.

According to the National Center for Complementary and Integrative Health (NCCIH), a division of the National Institutes of Health (NIH), yoga has been demonstrated to relieve stress, improve mental health and sleep, and reduce fall risk.[3] It helps reduce pain in the neck and knees, as well as reducing headaches. Practitioners are often motivated to adopt other healthy habits, leading to weight loss or reduced cravings for nicotine and ultra processed food.

I introduced intentional movement in my life through daily yoga practice. Since I do it at home, a morning practice inserts easily between brushing my teeth and getting dressed for the day. And I find practicing for twenty minutes every day with an on-demand class much easier than driving to a studio for an hour-long class twice a week. When I first started practicing yoga, I lacked the strength and agility for some of the poses. Initially, I felt like a giant jellybean rolling around on the mat, but my body got stronger over time. My yoga practice has had a profound impact on my health for several reasons.

With the emphasis on linking breath to movement, yoga requires sufficient focus to quiet the mental chatter. Also, as you know already, intentional breathing triggers relaxation of the nervous system. In yoga, we contract and release energy locks called *bandhas* to stimulate the flow of energy. The gentle stretching stimulates the flow of blood and lymph and dissipates morning stiffness. What kept me going in the beginning—and all these years later—is how alert and calm I feel after practicing. Skipping my morning yoga practice is as uncomfortable as not brushing my teeth.

Qigong

Associated with TCM, qigong developed in China over four thousand years ago. Qi (pronounced *chee*) refers to our life-force energy. Qigong practitioners learn to protect and consciously guide the movement of their qi to promote optimal health and healing.

The practice is similar to yoga in that it involves a series of movements linked to the breath. In addition, qigong emphasizes adequate sleep, proper nutrition, and stress management. The movements are intended to promote flow of energy through the meridians. As we learned earlier, the primo vascular system offers anatomical evidence that these meridians exist and deliver life-sustaining substances throughout our body.

The health benefits of Qigong have not been widely studied; however, the NCCIH lists blood pressure, chronic heart failure, chronic obstructive pulmonary disease (COPD), knee pain, reduced cognitive ability, cancer, substance abuse, balance difficulty, Parkinson's disease, and fibromyalgia as conditions that appear to benefit from a regular qigong practice. According to the National Qigong Association (NQA), benefits also include improved coordination, flexibility, strength, respiration, circulation, and pain management, as well as balancing the immune and nervous systems. Despite the lack of clinical studies, the fact that Qigong has been practiced for thousands of years is a testament to its effectiveness. According to NCCIH, the risk of injury while practicing qigong is low.

As with yoga, seek out an instructor who offers tips for proper alignment. The NQA has an online directory of certified and professional members.

Tai Chi

Tai Chi is a form of Qigong. Both are rooted in TCM and focus on the life force energy, or chi. Both involve slow, meditative movements coupled with the breath. Some of the movements in Tai Chi are more complex, as it is intended as practice for developing the physical abilities required in martial arts.

Tai chi has been more widely studied than qigong. According to a 2016 systematic review of clinical trials published in *The Canadian Family Physician*, there is excellent evidence that tai chi is beneficial for preventing falls, improving the symptoms of osteoarthritis, COPD, and Parkinson's disease, and strengthening cognitive ability in older adults.[4] The review also provides good evidence that tai chi is beneficial for depression, cardiac and stroke rehabilitation, and dementia.

Walking

Walking is the oldest, simplest, and most popular exercise on this list. It requires no special equipment or gym membership, and odds are you already know how to do it! In intentional walking, keep the back erect and the arms relaxed, allowing them to swing gently by your sides. Remember to breathe slowly and deeply. Strive for an even stride; some wearable devices track the symmetry of your steps. Walk as briskly as you can without becoming breathless. The American Heart Association recommends beginners aim to walk for ten to fifteen minutes at a time, gradually working up to twenty-minute intervals for a total of 150 minutes per week.

The benefits of walking are widely accepted. Brisk walking increases our metabolism, so we store less energy as fat. A Harvard study involving 12,000 participants concluded that walking for an hour a day reduced the effects of thirty-two obesity-promoting genes by 50 percent.[5] It reduces arthritis pain by lubricating the joints and strengthening the surrounding muscles. Walking after a meal may reduce glucose spikes.

Some people like to listen to music or talk on the phone while walking, but a distraction-free walk gives you time to practice focusing on what is important. Stay safe by keeping distractions to a minimum when walking outdoors. Lower the volume on your headphones and pay attention to your surroundings. Consider investing in reflective clothing so drivers can see you in low-light situations.

If the area where you live is not conducive to walking, try walking indoors with an online coach. I like to practice online with a physical trainer who interjects simple dance steps to break up the monotony of walking in place. An online program is also a great alternative when extreme temperatures or wet weather interferes with your walking regimen.

Building Strength

Regaining the fitness level I needed to carry the vacuum cleaner up the stairs unaided required increasing my physical strength. Since regular gym visits aren't sustainable given my schedule, I practice at home with a pair of free weights.

Working with weights or resistance bands increases the proportion of lean mass in our body, thereby increasing our metabolism. Strengthening muscles also strengthens our bones, counteracting the gradual bone loss that begins in middle age. The activities of daily living—such as carrying groceries or cleaning our home—are more accessible when we are physically strong.

If you are new to resistance training, I highly recommend consulting with a personal trainer to learn proper form and avoid injury.

The Importance of Hydration

Introducing intentional movement into your life will increase your body's need for fluid. Our hydration requirements vary depending on gender, age, weight, activity level, medications, and the weather. The current recommendation is nine cups a day for women and thirteen cups for men.

Getting enough fluid does not require gulping down copious amounts of water. The moisture in food counts toward our total fluid intake. Fresh produce has a particularly high water content.

Symptoms of dehydration include thirst, headache, dizziness, fatigue, dry mouth or skin, reduced sweating or urination, dark-colored urine, and constipation. Sometimes, hunger is your body's way of letting you know that it needs more moisture. According to research conducted by NIH, chronic dehydration increases your risk for heart failure, diabetes, chronic lung disease, and dementia.[6]

By now, you understand the consequences of consuming fruit juice and beverages with added sugar. Water is our best choice, but plain tea, black coffee, and unsweetened flavored water are other options.

As with other healthy habits, we are more likely to practice them if they are incorporated into our routine. Some people fill a large water bottle in the morning and carry it with them with the goal of emptying it by the end of the day. Are you sufficiently hydrated? If not, what are your strategies to increase your fluid intake?

The Need for Rest

In his book *Celebrating Silence,* Sri Sri Ravi Shankar says, "Wisdom is knowing when to have rest, when to have activity, and how much of each to have."[7] During restorative sleep, our body redirects energy to cellular growth and repair. It keeps our systems functioning at their best.

While we sleep, the glymphatic system clears toxins from our brain. Researchers have discovered correlation between sleep deprivation and neurodegenerative disease. Lack of sufficient rest also appears to affect metabolism. According to Peter Attia, MD, author of *Outlive,* one night of poor sleep can alter how our body manages glucose levels the following day.[8]

Over time, insufficient sleep raises our risk of cardiovascular disease, Type 2 diabetes, obesity, and even death. The CDC estimates that each year, as many as 6,000 fatal vehicle accidents are the result of drowsy drivers.

An extensive review conducted by the Physical Activity Guidelines for Americans Advisory Committee in 2022 found strong evidence that physical activity improves sleep quality in healthy individuals.[9] In addition, they found moderate evidence that physical activity also improves sleep for people with insomnia and obstructive sleep apnea. Types of exercise practiced in the studies included walking, tai chi, yoga, resistance training, and aerobics.

A systematic review of twenty-three studies published in *Cureus* in 2023 concluded that gentle to moderate exercise shortened the time required to fall asleep and improved overall sleep quality.[10] According to the National Sleep Foundation, people who exercise in the morning sleep longer and spend 75 percent more time in restorative sleep cycles. Vigorous exercise less than two hours before bedtime, however, can make it harder to fall asleep.

Chronic anxiety is a major contributor to sleep issues, as a brain on high alert impedes our body's ability to relax. Practicing techniques like Intentional Breathing and the Infinity Technique on a regular basis builds resilience to the stress response, making sleep more accessible to us. Intentional movement is another way to purge stress response chemicals and regulate melatonin levels and circadian rhythms, leading to longer, deeper, and more restful sleep.

The Dangers of Sitting

Whenever we are moving, we aren't sitting. Sitting for extended periods of time impedes blood flow in our legs, increasing risk for blood clots and varicose veins. The less we walk, the more the large muscles of the hips, core, and legs weaken, setting us up for a vicious downward spiral as we avoid activities that involve extended walking or standing due to the added effort required. Hunching over a desk for long periods puts pressure on the spine, leading to back, shoulder, and neck pain. Excessive sitting is associated with digestive issues, lowered metabolism, weight gain, and diabetes. Some studies have linked excessive sitting with increased risk of fatal diseases, including cancer.

Sitting for long periods may be unavoidable for you. It is estimated that over 80 percent of modern jobs are performed seated. Even if you manage to squeeze in a cardio class before work, it appears that the health benefits of regular workouts are negated if we sit for more than eight hours a day. Desks that convert to a standing position may help, but our body needs more than standing in one place.

A 2023 study in the journal *Medicine and Science in Sports and Exercise* reported that participants had lower blood pressure and glucose levels when they broke up long periods of sitting by walking for up to five minutes every hour.[11] Periodic breaks also boost productivity by providing a mental rest.

According to an article published in *Nature Medicine* in 2022, analysis of data from 25,000 users of wearable devices over seven years indicated that three brief periods of vigorous activity lasting one to two minutes each day lowered mortality risk by 38–40 percent and risk of cardiovascular disease by nearly 50 percent, even if people didn't engage in regular exercise.[12] The study defines vigorous activity as walking fast or climbing stairs.

The Two-Minute Stretch Technique

This short exercise is designed to insert movement into long periods of sitting. Set an alarm on your phone or wearable device to remind you to stand every sixty minutes and move your body. Follow the steps below or practice along with me using the video in the online companion.

1. Begin with both feet flat on the floor, shoulder-width distance apart. Soften your knees slightly while still maintaining an erect posture, with your shoulders directly above your hips and your tailbone tucked under. Raise your shoulders up toward your ears before dropping them down and back.
2. While inhaling deeply, raise your arms out and above your head. If you can, rise up on your toes as you inhale. Exhale slowly while allowing your arms to drift back down to your sides and your heels lower to the floor. Repeat twice.
3. Stretch both arms out straight in front. Cross your right arm over your left, interlock fingers and bring hands down and in toward your chest as in the Pretzel Technique.
4. Push your interlocked hands away from your body while dropping your chin slightly. Round your back, allowing your shoulder blades to stretch away from each other. Hold for a few seconds. Then release the interlock and repeat the exercise on the other side by crossing your left arm over your right.
5. Place your hands on your hips. Keeping your hips facing forward in the same position, slowly rotate your chest to the right and pause for a few seconds. Rotate slowly in the opposite direction. Repeat again in each direction.
6. March slowly in place, raising your knees as high as you comfortably can. As you raise each knee, try to tap it with the opposite hand while still maintaining an upright posture. It's okay if you cannot lift the knee high enough to tap. Just do the best you can without hunching forward.

The Remarkable Power of the Heart

While it may speed up with exertion or slow down during sleep, we perceive the human heartbeat as the steady tick-ticking of a metronome. In reality, though, we are energetic beings in constant flux.

Instead of pumping away mindlessly, a healthy heart constantly responds to fluctuations in our body and the environment. Scientists call this our heart rate variability (HRV). Experiments conducted by researchers at the HeartMath Institute indicate that a high HRV correlates with improved bodily functions (such as breathing), mental processes (such as problem-solving) and our emotional regulation. Although we cannot detect these minuscule variations—which are only fractions of a second long—there are devices that offer a glimpse into how our heart is performing.

Feelings such as anger or frustration, for example, cause the heart to beat in a rigid staccato, producing an erratic HRV pattern reminiscent of spiky white-capped waves on a stormy sea. Under the command of a rigid heartbeat, our body strains to function, like an orchestra without a conductor to keep the musicians in sync. One aspect of our nervous system is attempting to surge forward while another aspect is pushing back—similar to driving a vehicle with the parking brake engaged. Over time, the strain manifests as disease.

When we focus on feelings of appreciation or gratitude, however, our HRV waveform smooths out like gentle waves caressing the beach. Other psychophysiological aspects, including respiration, blood pressure, and brain waves, synchronize with the heart in a flowing dance. Our entire being comes into a state of wellness that the HeartMath Institute calls *coherence*.

At first, it seemed counterintuitive to me that a consistent heartbeat length represents disordered functioning. But, just as a flexible tree can bend with the wind instead of break, we are better equipped to deal with challenges when our heart adjusts its rhythm in tune with the circumstances.

A high HRV is associated with cardiovascular fitness, clear thinking, and resilience to stress. With our nervous system flexing in harmony with the heart, we can perform tasks with ease. The doorways to creative insight and intuition open wide. Not only does the ability to intentionally raise your HRV improve your own emotional self-regulation, but it can also stimulate coherence in a fussy toddler, irritated boss, or other people nearby. In one experiment, the systems of unwitting participants became coherent when fellow participants intentionally raised their own HRV.

Practices to improve HRV include intentional breathing, adequate sleep, and proper nutrition. Moderate exercise such as walking or yoga are also beneficial, although regular intense exercise has been shown to lower HRV.

The Heart-Focused Breathing Technique

The HeartMath Institute offers several techniques to improve HRV, including heart-focused breathing.

1. Begin with the Intentional Grounding Technique, which includes a few moments of Intentional Breathing.
2. Focus your awareness in the area of your heart. Placing one or both hands over your heart chakra may help you focus your attention in this area.
3. Bring to mind someone or something for which you are grateful—perhaps a loved one, a pet, or a fortunate circumstance.
4. Allow your heart to fill with gratitude.
5. As you continue to practice Intentional Breathing, imagine your heart opening wide and bubbling over with unconditional love for yourself and others.

Some biofeedback devices calculate our HRV so we can get real-time feedback while we practice techniques that promote coherence. These devices are widely available for personal use.

They monitor our heart rate at the earlobe, wrist, chest, or thumb. Studies indicate that HRV biofeedback training helps mitigate symptoms of depression and post-traumatic stress. One study found that just five sessions of HRV biofeedback training helped healthcare workers recover from the stress of caring for COVID-19 patients.

How to Move Your Body

In this chapter, we explored the health benefits of movement to reduce stress, improve sleep, and avoid the dangers of sitting for long periods. Strategies to integrate movement into our day include exercising in short segments and trying gentle exercises we can practice at home. Raising our HRV improves our overall health. We learned three new techniques: the Blowout, the Two-Minute Stretch, and Heart-Focused Breathing. Here are some key tips for moving your body:

1. Make intentional movement a habit by selecting five- to ten-minute time slots to integrate movement into your daily routine. Choose a movement that is compatible with your schedule and activity level. Use the Technique Practice Tracker sheet in the back of the book to document your experience.
2. Use your journal to explore how your mindset might be keeping you from being more active.
3. To overcome internal resistance to intentional movement, refer back to the Readiness Assessment at the beginning of the book.

4. Practice techniques like The Focuser and mental rehearsal to facilitate change.
5. Practice techniques like Intentional Breathing and Tracing Infinity to improve your sleep by reducing the effects of stress.
6. If you have to sit most of the day, set an alarm on your phone to remind you to get up and move for ten minutes every hour. You could walk around your workspace, climb the stairs, or practice the Two-Minute Stretch. Print out the Intentional Movement Practice Tracker in the back of the book to log your progress.
7. Practice the Heart-Focused Breathing Technique. We will come back to it in the next chapter.
8. Visit the HeartMath Institute's website to learn more about HRV.
9. Retake the Chronic Anxiety Self-Assessment. Log your score in the Self-Assessment Tracker to monitor changes in your stress level over time.

ELEVEN
INTENTIONAL RELATIONSHIPS

I intend to connect with other people.

THAT SATURDAY I was handing out brochures about Healing Touch and other wellness topics at a local health fair. As I greeted the woman approaching my table, she began peppering me with nutrition questions. She would let me say only a few words before she would shake her head side-to-side, signaling her disapproval with my response. Glancing down at the materials on display, she pointed to my handout on carbs. "Well, at least you know the difference between simple and complex sugars," she sighed.

Old me would have felt offended and probably a teensy bit (okay, a lot) angry. But I realized that her animosity had nothing to do with me; something else had already lit her flame. So, I got curious instead. Breathing with intention, I focused my attention on her. I imagined a stream of open-heart energy flowing from my heart chakra to hers as her low-vibe energy drained out through her feet. She sighed and visibly relaxed. Sensing the energetic currency of my attention, she chatted amiably with me for at least ten minutes before moving on to the next table.

In this chapter, we will apply what we have been learning and practicing to make not only ourselves, but also the world, a better place. We will learn how to expand our inner self-healing into our connections with other people. Whether family members, close friends, or random strangers, we can uplift others by being our calm, grounded, and coherent selves. Intentional relationships are about realizing that all people are interconnected.

No One Is an Island

Speaking to the importance of community in 1624, John Donne declared, "No man is an island." Modern-day research confirms what Donne inherently knew—that we are more connected than we realize.

The Six Degrees of Separation theory states that each of us is connected to every other person on the planet by an average of six relationships. In other words, you are connected to all the friends of your friends through two relationships: the relationship you have with your friend, plus the relationship between your friend and their friends. According to the theory, you can trace connections to anyone through six or fewer connections, or hops.

Originally theorized by social psychologist Stanley Milgram in the 1960s, Microsoft conducted an experiment that revised the number of connections to 6.6 in 2006. The proliferation of social media appears to have lowered the number of connections. Five years after Microsoft's experiment, Facebook analysis found that 92 percent of users were connected by no more than five relationships.

Since meeting the photographer Platon in 2017, I can trace my connection to the dozens of world leaders and celebrities that he has photographed in just two hops. By reading my book, you are now only three connections removed from the past six U.S. Presidents, Putin, and Adele. But I believe that the theory is true with less-connected people we know, as well.

One morning, my bird-watching group ended our hike with breakfast at a nearby coffee shop. There were so many of us that the group could not all sit at the same table. I ended up with a couple I knew and a woman, Judy, who was joining us for the first time. As we chatted, it came to light that Judy had just relocated from Chicago, and it turned out her best friend was the husband's sister. Imagine—if we had sat at different tables, they would not have discovered their connection.

We are more connected to the rest of the world than we realize! The next time you are in a crowded place, remind yourself that—although you may not know how—you are connected to every stranger you see through fewer than seven relationships.

The importance of our interconnectedness becomes clear when we consider the health benefits of interacting with others. According to a research review compiled by Americorps, volunteering reduced age-related incidents of heart disease and mortality. Individuals with debilitating pain experienced a reduction in their symptoms when they volunteered to help others suffering from chronic pain. A 2023 survey conducted in Wisconsin concluded that "a positive sense of community is associated with a reduced reporting of depression, anxiety, and stress symptoms."[1]

In her work studying the power of intention, McTaggart has found that holding positive intentions for others has a mirror effect. According to her website, "After participating in Peace Intention Experiments, the participants' lives become more peaceful and loving, and in about a third of cases, they themselves get healed."

According to the U.S. Surgeon General's report "Our Epidemic of Isolation and Loneliness," published in 2023:

> Indeed, the effects of social connection, isolation, and loneliness on mortality are comparable, and in some cases greater, than those of many other risk factors including lifestyle factors (e.g., smoking, alcohol consumption, physical inactivity), traditional clinical risks factors (e.g., high blood pressure, body mass index, cholesterol levels), environmental factors (e.g., air pollution), and clinical interventions (e.g., flu vaccine, high blood pressure medication, rehabilitation).[2]

The desire for belonging is so strong that our survival instinct may prompt us to leave our native tribe in search of a more compatible community, or to pretend to agree with others to foster harmony within our existing group.

The Root chakra—associated with our sense of belonging and our place in society—is the only chakra that begins to develop before we are born. It functions best when we feel safe within our tribe. Anchored at the base of the spine and projecting downward toward the Earth, this chakra forms the base—or root—of our identity. Because of its foundational role, a balanced Root chakra facilitates our self-growth journey. We need to feel anchored in our connections with ourselves and others before we can truly flourish. Direct contact with the Earth, Intentional Grounding, and Intentional Movement can strengthen our Root chakra.

How Stress Affects Our Relationships

In *The Butter Battle Book*, Dr. Seuss tells the story of two communities bitterly divided over disagreements about how to spread butter on a slice of bread. The conflict escalates until one side develops a weapon that threatens to destroy them all.

Chronic anxiety makes us feel vulnerable. With our brain on

high alert, we constantly scan for threats. We become susceptible to othering—an "us versus them" mindset that can lead to dehumanizing groups of people based on their religion, ethnic background, political views, or even their approach to bread buttering. In extreme cases, we may romanticize the virtues of everyone in our "us" group while demonizing members of the "them" group to justify discriminatory, or even violent, behavior. Throughout history, othering has been used to pit groups against each other to further political agendas. The U.S. Civil War, the Japanese and Jewish concentration camps during World War II, and the "Troubles" in Northern Ireland are examples of violence arising from othering.

Unconscious bias is a form of othering residing so deeply within our mindset that we aren't aware it exists. It may have sprouted from social conditioning, personal experiences, or information from someone we trust, particularly at a young, impressionable age. Just as our brain fills in our peripheral vision with what it expects to be there, unconscious bias can trick us into making inaccurate assumptions about other people based on their outward appearance. It can diminish the quality of our relationships when we aren't seeing the other person as their authentic self. The practices of Intentional Focus and Intentional Mindset help us recognize when bias is distorting our perception. Project Implicit, a collaboration between Harvard University, the University of Virginia, and the University of Washington has free online quizzes to assess unconscious biases.

Stress can also lead to displaced anger or aggression, which is when we take out our frustration on an innocent bystander because we don't feel safe addressing the root cause of our emotions. The woman who confronted me at the health fair was expressing displaced anger, which I—in turn—could have taken out on someone else. But just because someone attempts to hand us a ball of low-vibe emotion does not mean that we have to accept it. We can metaphorically decline their "gift" with a firm but polite "no, thank you." As Eleanor Roosevelt said, "No one can make you feel inferior without your consent." By regularly practicing energetic self-care, we cultivate the skills to release low-vibe energy instead of passing it along to someone else.

I am on friendly terms with many people whose political persuasions are the polar opposite of mine. We get along because I refuse to let my flashlight of focus linger on our differences. That's a waste of energetic currency, as I cannot convince them to adopt my worldview any more than they can convince me to see things their way. Everyone's perspective is rooted in their personal experience, and we all have our blind spots.

Instead, I focus on areas of common ground—for they are always there if we make the effort to look for them. We all want to be healthy. We all want to feel safe, happy, and loved. We all want to belong to a tribe of like-minded individuals. And, I believe, we are all lit by an intangible spark of life that originated from the same flame.

Poet Maya Angelou points out that people remember how we make them feel more than what we say or do. Whether spending time with a long-term acquaintance or someone I just met, I train my flashlight of focus on them. We all notice someone's outward appearance—their clothing, grooming, mannerisms, and so on. Our attention skims over them much like I scanned the restaurant during my lunch with Janet. But if we stop there, our brain will fill in the missing bits based on assumptions.

Paying undivided, nonjudgmental attention to someone is mutually rewarding. In my experience, people tend to open up like a morning glory greeting the sunrise. I can't tell you how many times strangers have shared intimate stories before suddenly stopping to confess sheepishly, "I don't know why I am telling you all this." We both leave our encounter basking in the warmth of genuine connection with another human being.

Practice looking beyond people's gender, skin color, age, and political views. Tune in to their energy. What is the frequency of their biofield? What thoughts and emotions are they broadcasting? Get curious about why they think what they think. Ask questions and listen to their answers with an open heart. What does it reveal about their mindset? What does your reaction to them say about yours?

The Metta or Loving Kindness Meditation

This meditation has ancient origins in Buddhism. Because it was originally written in Sanskrit, the English translations vary—but they all follow the same format of sending compassion in ever-widening circles until we are radiating unconditional love to all life on the planet. The meditation begins with sending love to ourselves, because self-love is a prerequisite to authentically loving others. I find this meditation extremely effective at raising our vibe to a level approaching enlightenment. There is a recorded version of the mediation available in the online companion.

1. To begin, find a comfortable position, either sitting or lying down. As we do in Heart-Focused Breathing, practice Intentional Breathing while imagining your heart opening wide.
2. Say aloud or to yourself:

> May I be well, happy, and peaceful.
> May I be safe.
> May I be healthy and whole.
> May I always meet with success.
> May I also have the wisdom, courage, patience, and determination to meet and overcome inevitable difficulties, problems, and failures in life.

3. Bring to mind the people closest to you, such as family members and close friends. Say aloud or to yourself:

May they be well, happy, and peaceful.
May they be safe.
May they be healthy and whole.
May they always meet with success.
May they also have the wisdom, courage, patience, and determination to meet and overcome inevitable difficulties, problems, and failures in life.

4. Bring to mind your acquaintances—people you see on a regular basis such as friends and coworkers. Repeat the affirmations from step 3.
5. Bring to mind people you see occasionally and do not know very well—perhaps people who live in your neighborhood or work at a store you frequent. Repeat the affirmations from step 3.
6. Extend your focus to people who are suffering—they could be imprisoned, sick, cold, hungry, or grieving. Repeat the affirmations from step 3.
7. Radiate compassion to people with whom you have a contentious relationship, realizing that we all want to experience joy in life. Repeat the affirmations from step 3.
8. Now extend loving kindness to all life on the planet. Repeat the affirmations from step 3.

How Our Mindset Affects Our Relationships

Abby was upset that her friend, Mike, had not texted her back. "Obviously, he is ghosting me." she fumed. "That may be true," I agreed, "but there could be other reasons that you haven't heard back from Mike yet." The alternatives I rattled off included Mike being sick or injured, having been called away unexpectedly for a family emergency, having been assigned an urgent project at work, or dealing with an issue such as a car in the shop or a broken refrigerator. It was also possible that Mike's jealous girlfriend had deleted Abby's text before Mike saw it. Perhaps Mike had received Abby's text but didn't realize she expected an immediate response. I suggested that Abby reach out to Mike again with a casual, "Hey—how are you?" But Abby remained adamant that their friendship was over.

Although we may not be consciously aware of them, we all have expectations about how people should conduct themselves. These expectations evolve from our beliefs, values, personal experiences, and other mindset components. Relationship problems can often be traced to mismatched expectations. Abby expected a timely response, so she decided that their friendship was over when Mike still hadn't texted back days later. My friend Scot told me that his wife left him because he "didn't love her enough." He was genuinely perplexed because he viewed his behavior toward her as very loving.

One way to close the gap between expectations and reality in a relationship is to try to convince the other person to change into the person we want them to be. This approach rarely works, however.

A more effective approach is to examine ourselves. When we do the work to excavate our mindset, we can open the doors to understanding our expectations. Begin by clarifying your unmet expectations—an exercise best done in writing. Describe how you wish the other person behaved. For example, Abby expects Mike to text her back within a few hours. Perhaps Scot's wife expected him to help with the housework so she would have more free time on the weekends.

Then ask yourself, "Where does this expectation come from? What beliefs, values, or other mindset components created this expectation? Is this expectation in my best interests?" You may find that your expectations need adjusting. Or you may decide that the relationship needs to change, as I did with Lori when I realized that she had no qualms about lying to get her way.

Abby had yet to recover from a painful end to a long-term friendship years before. She had internalized the belief that "people leave, so it is better to leave them before they leave you." At the first hint that Mike wasn't prioritizing their friendship, she decided to end it.

Adopting a growth mindset empowers us to adjust our expectations when we decide that they need to change. As I shared earlier, I am a recovering perfectionist. I used to feel annoyed with people who produced sloppy work products. Once I investigated my mindset, however, I realized that perfectionism was not the asset I imagined it to be, and I released it.

This is not to imply, however, that we should always adjust our expectations to align with the other person's. Sometimes, it is the relationship that needs to change. I ended my friendship with Lori because I was unwilling to release the expectation that people should not lie to get what they want. Perhaps Scot and his wife would have come to a similar impasse in their marriage. Or maybe they would have found a way to align their expectations or to stay together despite the mismatch. Unfortunately, their marriage ended because they lacked the tools to figure it out.

To what extent could mismatched expectations be at the root of your relationship challenges? Grab your journal and use the Mind the Gap prompts in the back of this book to explore mismatched expectations and what you will do to address them.

Reframing Victory

In *The Art of War,* ancient Chinese military strategist Sun Tzu states that success is not the defeat of one's enemy but avoiding armed conflict in the first place. "The greatest victory is that which requires no battle."[3]

If we look below the surface of any divisive issue, such as gun control or abortion, we find different beliefs, values, personal experiences, and other mindset components. Too often, however, we engage in a tug-of-war over who is right without diving into *why* we think what we think. In our rush to "other" people with differing opinions, we neglect to ask ourselves, "What do they know that I don't? Where are my blind spots?" Finding common ground on an issue requires understanding not only our own mindset, but also the mindset of others. As Sun Tzu says, "If you know the enemy and know yourself, you need not fear the result of a hundred battles." Try these four steps the next time you find yourself at odds with someone.

1. Listen for Understanding

It's important to remain calm, grounded, and shielded while discussing a contentious topic with others. With regular practice of the Intentional Breathing, Intentional Grounding, and Energetic Shield techniques, you will be able to prepare yourself in seconds.

As the other person expresses their opinion, listen attentively to what they are saying. You will need to remember their main points for the next step. If your brain is composing retaliatory remarks, then you aren't paying close enough attention.

2. Summarize Key Points

When the other person finishes speaking, summarize your understanding of their main points. Maintain a neutral tone and resist the urge to scoff or roll your eyes. Simply restating your understanding of what they said does not mean that you agree—it just shows them that you were paying attention.

Ask the other person whether they agree that you summarized their perspective accurately. Ask something like, "Did I get that right?"

3. Move Forward or Go Back

Now this is where the discussion can go in different directions. Ideally, they will exclaim "Yes—you got it!" in which case you can move forward to the next step.

But they might reiterate their perspective. Perhaps they aren't satisfied with your summary, or they weren't listening to you. Either way, repeat the first two steps until they agree that you have summarized their viewpoint accurately.

True story—I have watched people go at each other with so much vitriol (and so little listening) that they didn't realize that they were saying the same thing. I confess that it was kind of fun to say, "You know you guys are vehemently agreeing with each other, right?"

4. List Areas of Agreement and Explore Differences

List areas where your perspectives overlap. You could say, "I agree with you that _____ [list areas of agreement]." Establishing common ground with other people feels reassuring to both parties. Not only does it validate our viewpoint, but a shared perspective also helps us both feel safe and connected.

Once people feel heard and understood, they may be ready to listen to your perspective, but that doesn't always happen. If they seem open, describe where your opinions diverge and explain why you disagree with theirs. You could say, "I am not on board with your perspective about X because I was raised to _____ [describe your mindset.]" Or you could say, "I am not on board with your perspective about X because, in my experience, _____ [describe your experience]."

Ideally, they will mirror your behavior from earlier by restating their understanding of what you said. But if the interaction feels uncomfortable to them, they may react with anger. It's okay if they aren't ready for an open-hearted exploration of your differences. I think of it as planting seeds that may sprout at a later date. Remember to exercise compassion and patience.

Your power lies not in getting other people to see the world the same way that you see it; your power lies in being at peace with your understanding of the world regardless of whether others share your viewpoint. You may learn something from the exchange that inspires you to adjust your mindset or clarifies why you feel the way that you do. Regardless of what happens, you will leave the interaction with the benefit of insight. The hope is that they will, too.

When Our Emotions Are Not Our Own

Like viruses, emotions are contagious. Whether in-person or online, between two people or a crowd of thousands, the emotions of one person can infect others. Known as *emotional contagion*, the effect can be inspiring or destructive.

Even before we have the ability to speak, emotional contagion influences relationships that are key to our survival. Studies have shown that when a mother feels anxious, her infant exhibits the physiological symptoms of stress. By our first birthday, we adapt our behavior based on social cues; if mom is in a foul mood, babies respond with wariness. As we mature, this subconscious emotional sensitivity allows us to connect with a mate and the other members of our tribe.

The Emotional Contagion Scale (ECS) measures our predisposition to catching five emotions from others: sadness, fear, anger, happiness, and love. According to the ECS, you may be more susceptible to emotional contagion if you tend to cry at sad movies, tense up when you overhear other people arguing, or forget your troubles in the presence of a happy person.

The beauty of emotional contagion is that other people can "catch" our high-vibe emotions when we radiate our inner joy. The downside of emotional contagion is when low-vibe emotions spread—such as when a crowd of peaceful protesters erupts into a violent mob. There's a difference between tuning into someone else's vibes and absorbing them into our field.

When we see people hurting, we may be tempted to feel bad for them. We are only hurting ourselves, however, when we take on emotions that are oozing out of someone else's burden bag. If I were to get mad at Mike on Abby's behalf for not returning her texts quickly, I'd be dragging down my energetic vibe, while doing nothing to lessen her pain. If you want to help someone, give them the energetic currency of your focus instead. Allow them to express their emotions without trying to fix their situation or share their pain.

Likewise, when communities are suffering from the effects of climate disasters or war, grieving someone else's losses accomplishes nothing. A better response is to volunteer our time, donate to recovery efforts, or radiate loving kindness in their direction

The Energy-Clearing Technique

In Healing Touch training, we learn to ground ourselves before every session because when we attune with a client, some of their emotions seep into our field. At the conclusion of every session, we disconnect from the client's biofield before cleansing our own field of any residual energy still clinging to us.

Once, when working with a client hospitalized with a life-threatening condition, I sensed his pervasive dread. My eyes pricked with tears as the client's fear flowed into me. Being grounded enabled me to release the fear, although I intuited that he would not live much longer and he knew it.

Everyone should know how to clear other people's emotions from their field. Intentional Grounding and the Energetic Shield Technique are two ways to increase resistance to viral emotions, but sometimes infectious energy clings to us anyway.

The Energy-Clearing Technique filters out emotional contagion with a virtual net. Practice this technique periodically, in addition to when your emotions feel out of alignment.

1. Begin by lifting your arms above your head and

spreading your fingers wide. Imagine a net stretched between the fingers of each hand.
2. With fingertips pointed toward you, slowly draw your arms down both sides of your body while repeating to yourself, "I release anything that is not mine." Intend for your imaginary net to trap any extraneous emotions that don't belong to you.
3. When your hands reach your knees, sweep them outward and away from you and shake them off.
4. Repeat two more times or until your field feels clear.

If the low-vibe emotions are still with you, then they may be yours. Remember that the only way out is through. Regardless of the source, we want to release the emotion instead of suppressing it.

We All Are Connected

Native Hawaiians were aware of our energetic connections. When a disagreement arose between two members, everyone accepted responsibility for the disharmony in the community—no matter how small or unintentional their role. All the members participated in a communal reconciliation ceremony—the Ho'oponopono (pronounced *hoe-oh-poe-no-poe-no*).

This perspective represents a paradigm shift for a society that settles disagreements in court. For us, justice entails identifying the guilty party and dispensing appropriate punishment.

From a quantum physics perspective, however, communal accountability makes sense. The energy of our emotions radiates outward like virus molecules lingering in the air after a sneeze. Even if they did not originate with us, disspelling low-vibe emotions prevents the spread and maintains harmony.

Remember my manager, Jill, with the urgency addiction? She would exacerbate little issues in the workplace. At the time, I viewed her predilection for drama as strictly a "Jill problem."

But from the perspective of the Ho'oponopono teachings, my irritation with her behavior was contributing to the low-vibe atmosphere in the office. I didn't know about the Ho'oponopono at the time, but practicing it alone or with trusted colleagues could have shifted the energy and perhaps relieved Jill of her need to stir up drama.

The Ho'oponopono may be used to rectify a specific situation or as a regular practice. It's a powerful way to be part of the change that the world needs.

The Ho'oponopono Technique

The phrases may be stated in any sequence. As you recite these sentences, lean into the energy of the feelings they emote. Accept responsibility for the hurtful energy that we pass along from the field or our ancestors. Express regret for contributing to the disharmony in the world. Radiate unconditional love, recognizing that—just as one candle is used to light others—we are all enlivened by the same divine life-force energy. Appreciate the opportunity to transform hurtful energy, thereby healing the world and yourself in the process.

Follow the steps below or practice along with me using the video in the online companion.

1. To begin, find a comfortable position, either sitting or lying down.
2. As we do in the Heart-Focused Breathing Technique, practice Intentional Breathing while focusing your awareness in the area of your heart.
3. Bring to mind the situation you want to address.
4. Repeat aloud or to yourself the Ho'oponopono mantra until you feel the energy shift:

I'm sorry.
Please forgive me.
I love you.
Thank you.

How to Connect with Other People

In this chapter, we discovered the health benefits of connecting with others. As humans, our sense of safety depends on belonging to a group of like-minded individuals. Usually, relationship issues can be traced to mismatched expectations arising from our mindset. By examining our mindset, we can determine whether our expectations are accurate or due for an upgrade. Understanding the perspectives of other people is more practical than trying to convince them to see the world through our eyes. We learned how to distinguish our emotions from those we may have picked up via emotional contagion. Here are more tips for connecting with other people:

1. Write this chapter's intention (*I intend to connect with other people*) on a piece of paper and tape it to your bathroom mirror. Take a moment every morning to decide how you will practice the intention in the day ahead. At the end of the day, congratulate yourself for taking action to cultivate your personal power.
2. Remember that we are all connected in ways that we may never realize. Studies indicate that there is an average of six relationships between us and everyone else on the planet.
3. Practice Intentional Grounding and Intentional Movement to strengthen the Root chakra, which is associated with our sense of belonging.

4. Take the online quizzes available from Project Implicit to raise your awareness of your unconscious biases.
5. Practice the Metta meditation to tap into the vibe of unconditional love.
6. Practice paying undivided, nonjudgmental attention to family members, friends and strangers.
7. When conflicts arise, strive to understand why you feel the way that you do. Be open to adjusting your perspective, if appropriate.
8. Instead of attempting to convince others to see things your way (which rarely works), get curious about why they feel the way that they do.
9. Be aware of when you may have "caught" emotions from someone else. Use the Energy Clearing Technique to remove energy that is not yours.
10. Pick a point in your existing daily routine to practice The Ho'oponopono for two minutes at least twice every day. Use the Technique Practice Tracker sheet in the back of the book to track your progress until it becomes a habit.
11. Use The Ho'oponopono as appropriate to clear low-vibe energy circulating within a group. If they are receptive, teach The Ho'oponopono to others.
12. Retake the Chronic Anxiety Self-Assessment. Log your score in the Self-Assessment Tracker to monitor changes in your stress level over time.

TWELVE
LIVING THE EIGHT INTENTIONS

Congratulations! You made it to the end of the book! Take a moment to honor yourself for making time to take care of yourself and—by extension—the people who depend on you.

Like our skeleton supports our physical body, the eight intentions provide a framework for our life. Use them to set the tone for each day and guide your choices. But keep in mind that the intentions are not hard and fast rules. Each of us will embody the intentions in our own unique way.

Think back to when you first picked up this book. What did you hope to accomplish? To what extent have you been successful in achieving that outcome? How has practicing the intentions affected your health and relationships with yourself and others?

Review your scores from the Chronic Anxiety Self-Assessments. What was going on in your life when your anxiety level was low? How can you cultivate more of those circumstances?

There's a famous saying that "old habits die hard." By integrating the eight intentions into your existing routine, you allow them to become automatic behavior.

I begin every day focused on gratitude. Before I get dressed for the day, I take twenty minutes for intentional movement.

Whether I practice yoga or cardio, exercise releases stress chemicals from my bloodstream and raises my vibe. I break my fast with a high-fiber concoction of whole grains and fresh fruit. So, I automatically tap into six of the eight intentions every morning.

Then, throughout my day, I use Intentional Breathing to counteract the stress response. I redirect my focus with affirmations if Scenario Sally makes an appearance. If someone says or does something that I don't like, I rely on journaling to unpack why it bothers me and what I can learn from the experience. I focus on similarities with other people instead of differences.

The Intend Well Wheel Exercise

The Intend Well Wheel Exercise is an easy way to check in with ourselves periodically. This self-assessment tool ensures that you are balancing all eight intentions by assessing the degree to which you are practicing each of them. If you find that you are paying more attention to some intentions while ignoring others, implement strategies to bring your intentions back into balance. Instructions are in the back of the book as well as the online companion.

How to Live the Eight Intentions

Living the eight intentions is like strength training. Our muscles only stay strong as long as we exercise them regularly. Sometimes, life interferes with our well-established habits and, before we know it, our self-healing power is compromised. The following steps will help as you commit to living the eight intentions.

1. Review the tips at the end of every chapter.

2. Look for ways to integrate the eight intentions into your daily routine.
3. Pay attention to the thoughts you are thinking and emotions you are feeling.
4. Practice your favorite techniques until you can use them effortlessly when needed.
5. Revisit the Intend Well Wheel Exercise every so often to identify opportunities to strengthen your self-healing capability.

PART 3
SELF-EXPLORATION

THIRTEEN
WORKSHEETS AND EXERCISES

THE WORKSHEETS MENTIONED throughout the book are provided in this section. To make them easier to use, the free online companion includes full-sized (8.5 x 11) versions that you can print at home.

Scan the QR code below or visit *CarolynPitts.com/eightintentions* to download the online companion.

CHRONIC ANXIETY SELF-ASSESSMENT TOOL

Short-term bouts of anxiety are inevitable. Instead of seeking to eliminate anxiety, the goal is to learn how to manage it. I think of anxiety as a place I have to visit sometimes (like the dentist's office), but I don't have to live there. Anxiety becomes a health issue when it becomes our default state.

How to Use This Tool

1. For each symptom, place a checkmark in the column describing how frequently you experience it. If you never experience the symptom, leave the row blank.
2. Count the number of checkmarks in each column across all the pages.
3. Multiply the number of checkmarks in each column by one for Rarely, three for Some, and five for Often. Add these three numbers to get your Total Chronic Anxiety Score.
4. Review the score interpretation table that follows the assessment. Keep in mind that your score will fluctuate depending on what is happening in your life

but as you practice the techniques regularly, you should see an overall decline in your anxiety score.
5. Grab your journal and take some time to reflect on your reaction to this exercise.

- Did the results surprise you?
- Do you agree with the interpretation? Why or why not?
- Are you experiencing symptoms of chronic anxiety? Consider what triggers the stress response for you. Are there certain people or situations that elevate your stress level?
- How quickly do you recover from the stress response? Would you like to recover more quickly in the future?
- What did you learn from doing this exercise?

6. Turn to the Chronic Anxiety Self-Assessment Tracker. Enter today's date and score.
7. Schedule time on your calendar to retake the self-assessment in a few weeks.

Keep in mind that your score will fluctuate depending on what is happening in your life, but as you practice the techniques regularly, you should see an overall decline in your score.

Chronic Anxiety Self-Assessment

Symptom	Rarely	Some	Often
Lack of energy. It's hard to get out of bed or off the sofa.			
High blood pressure or reliance on medication to manage blood pressure.			
Difficulty focusing on tasks.			
Trouble weighing options and coming to a decision.			
Feeling overwhelmed.			
Feeling stuck and unsure how to move forward.			
Difficulty retaining information or learning something new.			
Tendency to dwell on what's wrong in your life or the world.			
General aches and pains or unexplained muscle soreness.			
Physical or emotional numbness.			
Easily angered or annoyed.			
Feeling vulnerable or unsafe.			
Craving sweet or salty foods.			
Preferring to stay home rather than go to social events.			

CHRONIC ANXIETY SELF-ASSESSMENT TOOL

Symptom	Rarely	Some	Often
Difficulty setting boundaries.			
Yelling or throwing things.			
Feeling critical of others. Why can't anyone do things the right way?			
Difficulty falling or staying asleep.			
Mean self-talk. Saying critical things about yourself.			
Frequently ill.			
Feeling jittery or unsettled.			
Dizziness.			
Unexplained cold hands or feet.			
Intestinal bloating or gas.			
Acid reflux, frequent burping, sour stomach.			
Weight gain.			
Feeling disconnected from or outside your body.			
Constipation.			
Uncomfortable with uncertainty.			
Doing things that you don't want to do to please other people.			
Dwelling on worst-case scenarios.			

Symptom	Rarely	Some	Often
Injuries or illnesses take longer to heal.			
Prone to injury.			
Unexplained pain.			
Total checkmarks in each column			
Number of checkmarks in **Rarely** _____ x 1 =			
Number of checkmarks in **Some** _____ x 3 =			
Number of checkmarks in **Often** _____ x 5 =			
Total Chronic Anxiety Score			

	How to Interpret Your Score
128–170	Consider what may be contributing to your elevated anxiety. If there is something specific that is weighing on your mind, you may want to focus on intentional release. Plan to practice tapping two or more times a day until the issue is less troubling.
85–127	You may want to focus on intentional resilience. Plan to practice at least two minutes of intentional breathing three or more times a day.
84–43	Your anxiety is well-managed but, there is room for improvement. You may want to reprogram your mindset through intentions.
42 or less	Congratulations! You're doing a great job managing your anxiety. You may want to focus on intentional nutrition, movement, and relationships.

CHRONIC ANXIETY SELF-ASSESSMENT TRACKER

Use this sheet to keep track of your score every time you complete the Chronic Anxiety Self-Assessment. Ideally, you will see your score decline as you integrate the Eight Intentions into your life, but there will always be times when circumstances become more challenging. For many of us, fight-or-flight becomes our default state without realizing it. Tracking your results over time will raise your awareness of how you are feeling.

Chronic Anxiety Self-Assessment Tracker

Date	Score	Notes

TECHNIQUE PRACTICE TRACKER

The energy medicine techniques are most effective when practiced every day, in addition to as needed to counteract the stress response. Choose a point in your existing routine to practice a technique. Use the Technique Practice Tracker to document your practice for seven straight days or until it becomes a habit.

How to Use the Technique Practice Tracker

1. Enter the day's date at the top.
2. Write down the name of the technique you practiced.
3. Circle the appropriate faces to record how you felt before and after each practice session.
4. There is space on each page for additional notes about your experience.

- When did you practice?
- What changes did you experience as a result?
- What circumstances made it easier or harder for you to practice?

5. At the end of seven days, grab your journal and reflect on your experience.

- Were you able to make time to practice twice every day? Why or why not?
- Was practicing the technique every day beneficial?
- How well did practicing every day fit into your routine?
- How did practicing for seven days affect your stress level?
- What challenges did you encounter?

Technique Practice Tracker

Today's date: _____

Technique: _____

Before Practice

😊 😐 😟 🙁 😠 😢

After Practice

😊 😐 😟 🙁 😠 😢

_____
_____
_____
_____
_____
_____
_____
_____

MINDSET MAP EXERCISE

Our mindset is shaped by our beliefs, values, personal experiences, social conditioning, self-identity, and information from sources that we trust. It determines how we perceive ourselves and the world around us, as well as guides our decision-making and how we behave in certain circumstances. Our physical, mental, and emotional health are impacted by our mindset.

Imagine you are studying an intricate sculpture at a museum. As you walk around the statue, it may look different from various angles, but it is still the same object. This exercise is designed to help you gain insight into your mindset by considering it from different angles. Although we will examine each mindset component individually, in reality these elements are tightly interwoven. Don't get too caught up in whether something is a belief, a value, or social-conditioning. All that matters is the personal insight that arises.

Limiting Beliefs

Review the common limiting beliefs listed in the table. Place a checkmark next to the beliefs that feel true to you. Feel free to add your own in the space provided.

Limiting Beliefs

	I'm not good enough.
	Mistakes are bad.
	My opinion doesn't matter.
	The world is a dangerous place.
	Everyone is only looking out for themselves.
	Other people's needs are more important than mine.
	Money is the root of all evil.
	I don't have a creative bone in my body.
	My parents didn't love me enough.
	No one cares what I think.
	If my partner really loved me, they would _____.
	The right partner will want to take care of me.
	I never get a break.
	Poor health is a natural part of the aging process.
	I'm not smart/attractive.
	I hate my body.
	My problems are my parents' (or someone else's) fault.
	I'm too young/old.
	I'm not lovable.
	When I achieve my goal (lose weight, meet the right person, get a better job), then life will be perfect.
	I don't know why I bother to try.

	I have to suffer to be successful.
	Nothing ever works out for me.
	It's not my fault because it runs in my family.
	Life isn't fair.
	I can't trust anyone.
	There's nothing I can do to change the situation.
	It's better just to go along to get along.
	I catch every virus that is going around.
	No one listens to me.
	Politicians can't be trusted.
	There's nothing special about me.
	A successful career means making a lot of money even if you hate your job.
	I don't deserve anything better.
	If I am true to myself people won't like me anymore.
	It is better to give than to receive.
	I need to solve my problems on my own.
	Asking for help is a sign of weakness.
	There's no point in trying if I'm not sure I will succeed.
	Success is measured in promotions.

Values

What are your values? Review the values in the list below and place a checkmark next to the ones that apply to you. Words can mean different things to different people. Feel free to clarify a value or add your own in the space provided.

Choose values that influence your behavior and decision-making. While you may admire many of the values listed, think of ways that you actively express them. For example, you may think generosity is a virtue, but if you cannot cite examples of when you donated time and/or money to others, it may not be one of your values.

Experience	Generosity	Fairness
Creativity	Frugality	Pleasure
Wealth	Stability	Education
Safety	Courage	Altruism
Assertiveness	Family	Self-sufficiency
Kindness	Community	Reliability
Sustainability	Independence	Equality
Flexibility	Knowledge	Autonomy
Consistency	Personal growth	Integrity
Loyalty	Achievement	Humility
Patience	Enjoyment	Freedom
Honesty	Accountability	Trustworthiness
Commitment	Forgiveness	Friendship

Use your journal to explore the questions in the following sections.

Personal Experiences

- List personal experiences that had a strong impact on you, perhaps even changed the direction of your life.
- How might those events have impacted your current mindset?

Social Conditioning

- Describe the tribe of your childhood. How were people expected to dress, behave, and interact? Were expectations different based on gender? Was your childhood tribe patriarchal? Did men make decisions for the group, or was power balanced between the sexes?
- How might the colors you wore and toys you played with reflect the gender expectations of your tribe? How does your tribe celebrate births, marriages, and deaths?
- Was there a coming-of-age ceremony?
- What are some of the customs or rules for engagement embraced by your native tribe, friend circle, or coworkers?
- Were you taught to be self-reliant or to rely on others to take care of you?
- Are you still adhering to rules of engagement that don't align with your current circumstances? What behaviors could get someone ousted from the tribe?
- Think about the ways you interact with the people in your various social circles. Do you ever feel compelled to adopt a persona that violates your beliefs or values?
- If so, why do you think that is?
- What action can you take to improve the situation?

Self-Identity

- How would you describe yourself to someone else? Do you focus on what you see as your strengths (I am a whiz in the kitchen), or do you apologize for what you see as your weaknesses (I stink at math).
- How accurate is your self-perception? Can you recall specific situations when you exhibited the traits that you attribute to yourself?
- How do your friends describe you?
- What would your boss and coworkers say about you?
- What role has personal experience and social conditioning played in shaping your sense of self?
- Do you have any secret dreams?
- Is there anything that you would like to do but haven't tried? Why or why not?
- Do you make things happen, or do things happen to you?
- Are you comfortable with how you see yourself, or do you have a list of things you want to change? Consider what qualities or behaviors irritate you. Could it be that they remind you of an aspect of yourself that you secretly reject?
- What's the tone of your inner dialogue? Do you criticize or reassure yourself when you make a mistake?
- How often do you compare yourself to others?

Who Do You Trust?

- Who do you trust?
- Why do you trust them?
- How do you stay in touch with current events?
- Why do you trust these news sources?

Mapping Your Mindset

Now let's tie these components together.

- How would you describe your mindset?
- Think of your closest friends. How is their mindset similar to yours? How is it different?
- Recall that thoughts and emotions are energy. What is the vibratory nature of your mindset? Are you primarily optimistic or pessimistic? Are you the hero, villain, or victim of your life story?
- How does your mindset affect your overall health? How does your mindset affect your interactions with others?

The components that shape our mindset are also subject to change. As we journey through life, new personal experiences will lead to shifts in our beliefs, values, and self-identity. We can let go of outmoded social conditioning that doesn't serve us.

- How does your mindset support or inhibit your personal growth?
- How does your mindset support or inhibit your physical, mental, and emotional health?
- Has your mindset remained steady since early adulthood, or has it shifted?
- Why do you think that is?

LIMITING BELIEFS EXERCISE

Select a limiting belief from the Mindset Map Exercise. Then use your journal to explore the following questions. Repeat for each limiting belief you identified.

1. What is the limiting belief?
2. How do your values support or contradict this belief?
3. Where did this belief originate? Can you recall specific life experiences that relate to this belief?
4. How might your upbringing have contributed to this belief?
5. How does this belief shape the way that you see yourself?
6. How does this belief influence the way that other people see you?
7. How does this belief influence who you trust?
8. How does this belief inhibit your personal growth?
9. Is this belief true and supportive for you now?
10. If not, what might be a more healthful belief to have instead?

AFFIRMATIONS EXERCISE

In this exercise, we will create your personal list of affirmations to help reprogram aspects of your mindset that are not serving you.

Refer back to your writing from the Life Lesson Journaling exercise. Let's choose an affirmation to reprogram your mindset around the behavior pattern that you want to change.

As you read through the following list of sample affirmations, pay attention to statements that resonate with you. Take special note of any affirmation that triggers a sensation of resistance. This is an opportunity to explore why the statement feels uncomfortable. Could it conflict with a subconscious "truth" from childhood?

- I am lean and healthy.
- Every molecule of my being is functioning perfectly.
- I am powerful and strong.
- Everything is always working out for me.
- I trust my inner guidance system.
- I release all emotion that is inconsistent with love.
- I choose to enjoy life.

- I radiate loving compassion to myself and everyone around me.
- I am worthy of love and respect.
- I create my own reality.
- Anything I can dream, I can become.
- My life is full of abundance and prosperity.
- I love and accept myself just as I am.
- My life flows freely.
- Ease is a sign I am on the right path.
- All is well in my world.
- I shower my blessings with gratitude.
- I am perfect just as I am right now.
- I forgive myself.
- My life is deeply satisfying.
- The universe loves, guides, supports, and protects me.
- I am safe.
- I choose to receive the blessings of the universe.
- I open my heart to love.
- I release my expectations of myself and others. I trust that what seems like setbacks are blessings in disguise.
- I deserve the best that life has to offer.
- I have a purpose.
- I can achieve anything by being in harmony with the universe.
- I am worthy.
- I own my power.
- I claim my strength.
- Inner peace is my birthright.
- Through my mindset I create my own reality.
- I choose to be my best. I am courageous.
- I am fluid and flexible.
- I accept life as it is.
- There is a lesson in every disappointment.
- I am here to learn and grow.
- I choose empowering thoughts and emotions.

- I release my fears for the future.
- I release my regrets from the past.
- I express my authentic self.
- I express myself freely and openly.
- It is safe to be me.
- I choose to change old patterns of behavior.
- I choose to believe that everyone is doing their best. Other people's opinions of me are none of my business.
- The sun shines brighter after a cloudy day. This too shall pass, and I will be stronger for the experience.
- I have plenty of time.
- It is safe to love.
- I am strong enough to be vulnerable.
- I nourish my body with healthful foods.
- I care for and respect my body. I am shielded from disease.

Keeping in mind what you learned about how your mindset contributes to behavior patterns that you want to change, write down at least five affirmations. Choose from the sample list or make up your own.

Put your affirmation list where you will see it and read it aloud twice a day for seven days. Use the Technique Practice Tracker to document your experience.

Affirmations are more than just words. What really matters is how we *feel* when we say them. The heart and mind execute your operating system in tandem like a dual core processor, and we want to reprogram both of them. Many of the programs directing your behavior were installed before you were old enough to choose your truth, but affirmations enable you to intentionally reprogram your mindset.

DAILY FOOD DIARY EXERCISE

Logging your food consumption for a day is a great way to ensure that you are eating a well-balanced diet. It can be a time-consuming practice, so it is not necessary to do it every day.

1. Begin by entering the date at the top.
2. Enter the recommended daily amount of protein, carbs, and fat for your age, gender, and activity level. The USDA offers a free online calculator here: www.nal.usda.gov/human-nutrition-and-food-safety/dri-calculator
3. Log everything that you eat for the day, using additional sheets as needed.
4. Refer to the product's nutrition label to calculate the amount of protein, added sugar, fiber, saturated fat, and unsaturated fat for each item. Note the serving size and enter the total amount of macronutrients based on the number of servings you ate. For products such as fresh produce that do not have a nutritional label, there are resources online you can use. The USDA maintains a database you can access here: https://fdc.nal.usda.gov/

5. At the end of the day, total the amounts in each column. Consider the following:

   - How does the amount of protein you consumed compare to the recommended amount?
   - How much added sugar did you consume compared to the total recommended amount of carbs? How does the amount of fiber you consumed compare to the recommended amount?
   - Did you eat more saturated or unsaturated fat? Calculate your total fat intake by adding the column totals for saturated and unsaturated fat. How does the amount of fat you consumed compare to the recommended amount?

6. Journal about what you learned from this exercise. What changes, if any, do you want to make going forward?

Daily Food Diary

Today's date: _____

	Protein	Carbs	Fiber	Fat
Recommended amount				

Food	# Srv	Protein	Carbs	Fiber	Sat Fat	Unsat Fat
Total amount						

DAILY PRODUCE TRACKER

Use your journal to record your experience eating at least five fruits and vegetables every day for seven days.

1. Enter the day's date.
2. Record how many servings of each type of produce you ate and how it was prepared—for example, raw, roasted, steamed or boiled.
3. Every day that you meet your goal of eating at least five servings of produce, celebrate your achievement by placing a sticker on the page.
4. Use your journal to answer the following questions.

- Were you able to enjoy at least five servings of produce every day? Why or why not?
- If not, what strategies can you employ to eat more produce?
- What changes (physical, mental, emotional) did you notice by eating more produce?
- Because you were eating more produce, did you eat less of other types of food?

INTENTIONAL MOVEMENT PRACTICE TRACKER

Sitting for long periods of time is associated with digestive issues, weight gain, and weakened muscles in our legs, hips, and core. It also increases the risk for blood clots, varicose veins, diabetes, and cancer.

Set a specific movement goal for seven consecutive days. Perhaps you will take a thirty-minute walk after dinner or practice qi gong for fifteen minutes every morning.

If you sit most of the day, one way to increase your activity level is to set an alarm on your phone to remind you to practice the Two-Minute Stretch Technique every hour.

Use your journal to record your experience.

1. Enter the day's date.
2. What types of movement did you practice and for how long?
3. Every day that you meet your movement goal, celebrate your achievement by placing a sticker on the page.
4. Use your journal to answer the following questions.

- Were you able to fulfill your movement goal every day? Why or why not?
- If not, what strategies can you employ to move more every day?
- What changes (physical, mental, emotional) did you notice by moving more?
- How did the extra movement affect your sleep?

MIND THE GAP EXERCISE

Use this set of journal prompts to clarify the source of relationship issues stemming from mismatched expectations.

1. From your perspective, what are the primary points of contention in your relationship?
2. From the other person's perspective, what are the primary points of contention in your relationship?
3. To what extent could mismatched expectations be at the root of your relationship challenges?
4. Where did your expectation(s) originate? It may be helpful to refer back to your Mindset Map.
5. Once you identify the source, consider whether your expectation is still valid for you. Why or why not?
6. If yes, what is the best course of action for all involved? If not, how could you reprogram your mindset using affirmations?

THE INTEND WELL WHEEL

Maintaining your personal power to heal involves continually investing the appropriate amount of effort into each of the eight intentions. But, sometimes the demands of daily living can redirect our attention.

This exercise helps to you determine when changes are warranted to rebalance how you are investing your valuable attention. There are no right or wrong answers. Each time you do the exercise your scores may shift based on what is happening in your life.

1. Each section of the wheel represents one of the eight intentions. As you review the statements in each category, consider how true they are for you based on how you feel today.
2. In each category, rate your level of satisfaction on a scale of 1 to 10. A score of 1 means there is space for improvement in that category. A score of 10 means you're fully satisfied with that category.
3. Turn to the image of the wheel and log your score by marking the corresponding ring.
4. Reflect on the following questions in writing.

- What did you learn from this exercise?
- Which intentions warrant more investment?
- What actions will you take this week to increase your score in these areas?

5. Schedule a date to repeat this exercise.

Resilience Score

Stress is an inevitable aspect of daily life. Resilience is our ability to diffuse our stress in healthful ways through intentional techniques such as deep breathing, grounding, movement, and tapping.

- I recover quickly when things do not go according to plan.
- I have a sense of control over my life.
- I practice techniques to increase my resilience to stress.
- My sleep is deep and restorative.
- I laugh easily and enjoy being me.

Vibrational Frequency Score

Humans are energetic beings vibrating at a frequency measured in hertz. High-frequency thoughts and emotions have a positive impact on our overall health. Consider whether the following statements are true.

- I feel safe expressing my authentic self.
- I give voice to my feelings in ways that respect others.
- I avoid burying or suppressing negative emotions.
- I chose uplifting music, books and movies.

Focus Score

Energy flows where attention goes. Focus is about directing our attention towards the things that matter the most to us. Consider whether the following statements are true.

- I am clear about my priorities.
- I dedicate significant energy to fulfilling my life purpose.
- I have an inner compass that guides my decision-making.
- I experience a sense of serenity.

Mindset Score

Our mindset influences how we see ourselves and the world around us. A growth mindset enables us to examine our assumptions and reactions as we learn about ourselves. Consider whether the following statements are true.

- I see challenges as opportunities for personal growth.
- I unearth and reprogram limiting beliefs.
- I regularly ask myself, "Why do I think that I think what I think?"
- I respond compassionately yet firmly to my inner critic.
- I am living in harmony with my values.

Release Score

Release involves letting go of regrets, resentments and other burdens that impede the ability to self-heal. Consider whether the following statements are true.

- I accept that no one is perfect, nor should they strive to be.
- I don't dwell on situations that I cannot change.
- I believe that forgiveness is a gift that I give to myself, not to the other person.
- I allow my energy to flow unimpeded by eliminating clutter in my environment.
- I resist the urge to condemn or fix other people.

Nutrition Score

Our eating patterns have a direct impact on our gut microbiome, brain health, body weight and chronic diseases such as cardiovascular disease and Type 2 diabetes. Consider whether the following statements are true.

- I consume five or more servings of fruits and vegetables every day.
- I limit foods high in sugar, white flour, and unpronounceable chemicals.
- I avoid red or processed meats such as bacon and deli meat.
- I rarely, if ever, consume sugary beverages such as fruit juice or soda.

Physical Activity Score

Physical activity is about more than working out at the gym or going for a run. It's about having the strength and vigor to perform daily tasks. Consider whether the following statements are true.

- I engage in activity that elevates my heart rate for 30 minutes at least three times a week.

- I regularly engage in activities that strengthen my muscles.
- I avoid sitting for more than an hour at a time.
- I can rise from a chair, walk up steps, carry groceries and balance on one leg with ease.

Relationships Score

Humans are social animals. Our degree of connection with others has a direct correlation to our overall well-being. Consider whether the following statements are true.

- I have a close trusting relationship with at least three people.
- I have a sense of belonging to a community.
- I can set and respect interpersonal boundaries.
- I socialize with others on a regular basis.
- I rarely feel lonely.

244 THE INTEND WELL WHEEL

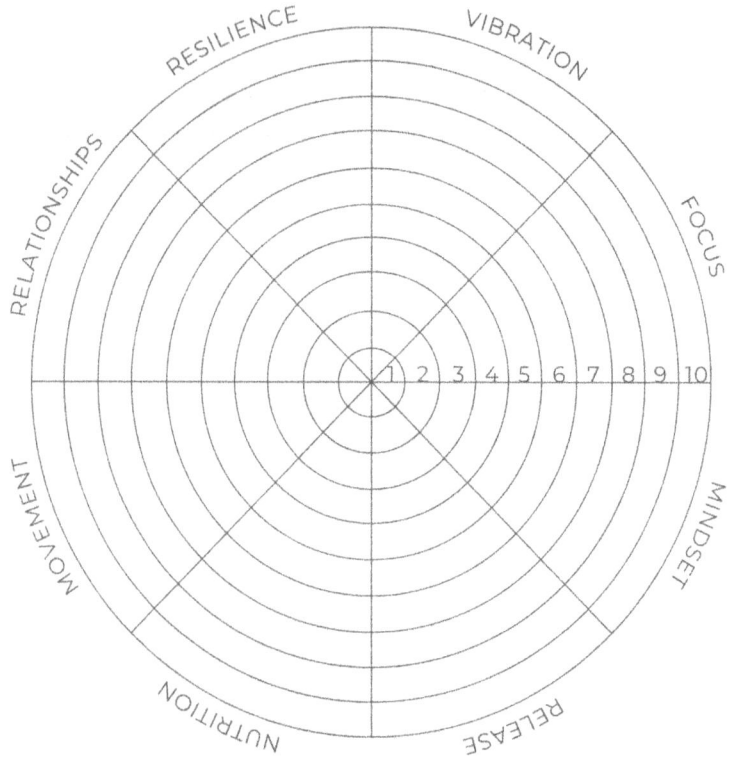

NOTES

1. All Healing is Self-Healing

1. Woolf, Steven H. "Necessary But Not Sufficient: Why Health Care Alone Cannot Improve Population Health and Reduce Health Inequities." *Ann Fam Med.* 2019 May;17(3):196-199. doi: 10.1370/afm.2395. PMID: 31085522; PMCID: PMC6827630
2. Kaplan RM, Milstein A. "Contributions of Health Care to Longevity: A Review of 4 Estimation Methods." *Ann Fam Med.* 2019 May;17(3):267-272. doi: 10.1370/afm.2362. PMID: 31085531; PMCID: PMC6827626.
3. Cox, Cynthia, Jared Ortaliza, Emma Wager, Krutika Amin. "Health Care Costs and Affordability." Kaiser Family Foundation. May 28, 2024. https://www.kff.org/health-policy-101-health-care-costs-and-affordability/?entry=table-of-contents-introduction

2. Ready, Set, Go!

1. Middleton KR, Anton SD, Perri MG. "Long-Term Adherence to Health Behavior Change." *Am J Lifestyle Med.* 2013 Nov-Dec;7(6):395-404. doi: 10.1177/1559827613488867. Epub 2013 Jun 14. PMID: 27547170; PMCID: PMC4988401.

4. Intentional Resilience

1. "Resilience." American Psychological Association. Accessed October 20, 2024. https://www.apa.org/topics/resilience

5. Intentional Vibes

1. Rubik B, Muehsam D, Hammerschlag R, Jain S. "Biofield Science and Healing: History, Terminology, and Concepts." *Glob Adv Health Med.* 2015 Nov 4 (Suppl):8-14. doi: 10.7453/gahmj.2015.038.suppl. Epub 2015 Nov 1. PMID: 26665037; PMCID: PMC4654789.
2. Chikly, Bruno & Roberts, Paul & Quaghebeur, Jörgen. "Primo Vascular System: A Unique Biological System Shifting a Medical Paradigm." *The Journal of the American Osteopathic Association.* 2016. 116. 12-21. 10.7556/jaoa.2016.002.
3. Hay, Louise. *You Can Heal Your Body.* Hay House, 1982.
4. Prestwood, Karen. "Energy Medicine: What Is It, How Does It Work, and What Place Does It Have in Orthopedics?" *Techniques in Orthopaedics.* 18 (2003). 46-53. doi: 10.1097/00013611-200303000-00009.

5. Hammerschlag R, Sprengel M, Baldwin AL. "Biofield Therapies: Guidelines for Reporting Clinical Trials." *Global Advances in Integrative Medicine and Health*. 2024;13. doi:10.1177/27536130231202501
6. Hendricks, Kimberly, and Kelley F Wallace. "Pilot Study: Improving Patient Outcomes with Healing Touch." *Advances in peritoneal dialysis. Conference on Peritoneal Dialysis* vol. 33,2017 (2017): 65-67.
7. Jain, Shamini et al. "Healing Touch with Guided Imagery for PTSD in returning active duty military: a randomized controlled trial." *Military medicine* vol. 177,9 (2012): 1015-21. doi:10.7205/milmed-d-11-00290
8. MacIntyre, Barb et al. "The efficacy of healing touch in coronary artery bypass surgery recovery: a randomized clinical trial." *Alternative therapies in health and medicine* vol. 14,4 (2008): 24-32.

6. Intentional Focus

1. How Much of the World Do You Really See? | Your Brain. PBS Learning Media. https://vpm.pbslearningmedia.org/resource/nvyb-sci-seebrain/how-much-of-the-world-do-you-really-see-your-brain/
2. Kreitz, Carina et al. "Inattentional Blindness and Individual Differences in Cognitive Abilities." *PloS one* vol. 10,8 e0134675. 10 Aug. 2015, doi:10.1371/journal.pone.0134675

7. Intentional Mindset

1. Alia J. Crum and Ellen J. Langer. "Mind-Set Matters: Exercise and the Placebo Effect." *Association for Psychological Science*. No. 18 (2). https://mbl.stanford.edu/sites/g/files/sbiybj26571/files/media/file/2007_exercise_mindset_crumlanger_psych_sci.pdf
2. Buchbinder, Rachelle. "Meniscectomy in Patients with Knee Osteoarthritis and a Meniscal Tear?" *The New England Journal of Medicine* 368, no. 18 (2013). doi:10.1056/NEJMe1302696
3. Landry M, Dornelles AC, Hayek G, Deichmann RE. "Patient Preferences for Doctor Attire: The White Coat's Place in the Medical Profession." *Ochsner J*, 2013 Fall;13(3):334-42. PMID: 24052762; PMCID: PMC3776508.
4. "Americans' trust in information from news outlets, social media." Pew Research Center October 17, 2024. https://www.pewresearch.org/newsletter/the-briefing/the-briefing-2024-10-17/#:~:text=New%20from%20Pew%20Research%20Center:%20Republicans%2C%20young,social%20media%20as%20from%20national%20news%20outlets.&text=In%20a%20new%20Center%20survey%2C%20adults%20under,(52%25)%20as%20from%20national%20news%20organizations%20(56%25).
5. Carter-Scott, Chérie. "Rules for Being Human." https://www.drcherie.com/media/rules-for-being-human-2/

8. Intentional Release

1. Hay, Louise. *You Can Heal Your Life*. Hay House, 1984.
2. Hawkins, David. *Letting Go: The Pathway of Surrender*. Hay House, 2012
3. Maté, Gabor. *When the Body Says No*. Alfred A. Knopf, 2003.
4. Hawkins. *Letting Go*.
5. Hawkins. *Letting Go*.
6. Hawkins. *Letting Go*.
7. "Thought Field Therapy: Algorithm Level Training Manual." *UK Institute of Thought Field Therapy and Callahan Techniques, Ltd*. 2014. https://www.thoughtfieldtherapy.co.uk/wp-content/uploads/2016/08/UKTFT-Algorithm-Manual.pdf

9. Intentional Nutrition

1. Delimaris, Ioannis. "Adverse Effects Associated with Protein Intake above the Recommended Dietary Allowance for Adults." *International Scholarly Research Notices*, 2013, 126929, 6 pages, 2013. https://doi.org/10.5402/2013/126929
2. Liu, Lanxiang et al. "Gut microbiota and its metabolites in depression: from pathogenesis to treatment." *eBioMedicine*, Volume 90, 104527 https://www.thelancet.com/journals/ebiom/article/PIIS2352-3964(23)00092-0/fulltext
3. Horta-Baas, Gabriel et al. "Intestinal Dysbiosis and Rheumatoid Arthritis: A Link between Gut Microbiota and the Pathogenesis of Rheumatoid Arthritis." *Journal of Immunology Research* vol. 2017 (2017): 4835189. doi:10.1155/2017/4835189 https://pubmed.ncbi.nlm.nih.gov/28948174/
4. Healthy Eating Plate. *Harvard Health Publishing*. https://www.health.harvard.edu/staying-healthy/healthy-eating-plate
5. "Soy and Cancer Risk: Our Expert's Advice." American Cancer Society. March 21, 2025. https://www.cancer.org/cancer/latest-news/soy-and-cancer-risk-our-experts-advice.html
6. "Soy-rich foods like tofu may help lower heart disease risk." American Heart Association. March 23, 2020. https://www.heart.org/en/news/2020/03/23/soy-rich-foods-like-tofu-may-help-lower-heart-disease-risk
7. Subali D, Christos RE, Givianty VT, Ranti AV, Kartawidjajaputra F, Antono L, Dijaya R, Taslim NA, Rizzo G, Nurkolis F. "Soy-Based Tempeh Rich in Paraprobiotics Properties as Functional Sports Food: More Than a Protein Source." *Nutrients*, Jun 1 2023;15(11):2599. doi: 10.3390/nu15112599. PMID: 37299562; PMCID: PMC10255641.
8. Ranasinghe, R. A. S. N., Maduwanthi, S. D. T., Marapana, R. A. U. J., "Nutritional and Health Benefits of Jackfruit (*Artocarpus heterophyllus* Lam.): A Review." *International Journal of Food Science*, 2019; 4327183, doi:10.1155/2019/4327183
9. Stapleton, Peta & Buchan, Craig & Mitchell, Ian & McGrath, Yasmin & Gorton, Paul & Carter, Brett. "An Initial Investigation of Neural Changes in Overweight Adults with Food Cravings after Emotional Freedom Tech-

10. Intentional Movement

1. "Exercise & Fitness." Harvard Health Publishing Sept 27, 2024. https://www.health.harvard.edu/topics/exercise-and-fitness
2. Monda, Vincenzo et al. "Exercise Modifies the Gut Microbiota with Positive Health Effects." *Oxidative Medicine and Cellular Longevity* (2017): 3831972. doi:10.1155/2017/3831972
3. "Yoga: Effectiveness and Safety." *National Center for Complementary and Integrative Health.* https://www.nccih.nih.gov/health/yoga-effectiveness-and-safety#:~:text=What%20are%20the%20health%20benefits,pain%20associated%20with%20knee%20osteoarthritis.
4. Huston, Patricia and Bruce McFarlane. 2016. "Health benefits of tai chi; What is the evidence?" *Canadian Family Physician* 62 no. 11 (2016): 881-890; https://www.cfp.ca/content/62/11/881
5. "5 surprising benefits of walking." Harvard Health Publishing. December 7, 2003. https://www.health.harvard.edu/staying-healthy/5-surprising-benefits-of-walking
6. Dmitrieva, Natalia I et al. "Middle-age high normal serum sodium as a risk factor for accelerated biological aging, chronic diseases, and premature mortality." *EBioMedicine* vol. 87 (2023): 104404. doi:10.1016/j.ebiom.2022.104404
7. Shankar, Sri Sri Ravi. *Celebrating Silence.* Arktos Media Ltd., 2021.
8. Attia, Peter. *Outlive: The Science and Art of Longevity.* Harmony, 2023.
9. Kline, Christopher E et al. "Physical activity and sleep: An updated umbrella review of the 2018 Physical Activity Guidelines Advisory Committee report." *Sleep medicine reviews* vol. 58 (2021): 101489. doi:10.1016/j.smrv.2021.101489
10. Alnawwar, Majd A et al. "The Effect of Physical Activity on Sleep Quality and Sleep Disorder: A Systematic Review." *Cureus* vol. 15,8 e43595. 16 Aug. 2023, doi:10.7759/cureus.43595
11. Duran, Andrea T et al. "Breaking Up Prolonged Sitting to Improve Cardiometabolic Risk: Dose-Response Analysis of a Randomized Crossover Trial." *Medicine and science in sports and exercise* vol. 55,5 (2023): 847-855. doi:10.1249/MSS.0000000000003109
12. Stamatakis, E., Ahmadi, M.N., Gill, J.M.R. et al. "Association of wearable device-measured vigorous intermittent lifestyle physical activity with mortality." *Nat Med* **28**, 2521–2529 (2022). https://doi.org/10.1038/s41591-022-02100-x

11. Intentional Relationships

1. Park, Eunice Y et al. "Sense of community and mental health: a cross-sectional analysis from a household survey in Wisconsin." *Family medicine and community health* vol. 11,2 (2023): e001971. doi:10.1136/fmch-2022-001971

2. "Our Epidemic of Loneliness and Isolation: The U.S. Surgeon General's Advisory on the Healing Effects of Social Connection and Community." U.S. Health and Human Services. 2023. https://www.hhs.gov/sites/default/files/surgeon-general-social-connection-advisory.pdf
3. Tzu, Sun. *The Art of War*. Shambhala Publications, Inc., 2001.

ACKNOWLEDGMENTS

Writing is a solitary activity, but transforming writing into a book is a collaborative effort. My deepest gratitude for the support I received along the way.

This book would not be possible without the benefit of my personal healing journey, which began when energy medicine entered my life. Thanks to Janet Mentgen for developing the Healing Touch program, and to my instructors Marilyn Stulb, Jean Pruett, and Walle Adams-Gerdts. Thanks, also, to Carol Komitor for developing and teaching the Healing Touch for Animals program.

Initially, I ignored the nudge to write a book. What did I know about publishing? But then the invitation to Hay House's Authorpreneur program arrived. Thanks to Reid Tracy, Kelly Notaras, Christa Gable, and the rest of the team for teaching me the ropes. The encouraging feedback on my book proposal gave me the confidence to keep going during the months that writing felt like a slog through deep, wet snow.

A professional editor enables a writer to see the book through the eyes of future readers. Thanks to the team at KN Literary Arts, particularly Marley Lynn and Nirmala Nataraj, for your invaluable frankness and supplying the thread so I could reinforce weak stitches. My deep appreciation also to eagle-eyed Leslie Wilson for tightening all the bolts and applying the final polish prior to takeoff.

When I began this book journey, my lifelong creativity did not extend to the written word. Writing was a unfamiliar craft that required developing new muscles. Thanks to Allegra Huston and James Navé for teaching my rational mind how to tango with creativity through the Imaginative Storm *Write What You Don't Know* course. Thanks also to my writing buddies in the Prompt of the Week workshops. Your creativity inspired me to reach deeper into my own.

Lively fellow travelers add enjoyment to shared adventures. Thanks to the amazing women of the Spiritual Writers Accountability Group: Donna Fado Ivery, Jennifer Corinna, Sandy Myodo Gougis, Joni Lamb, Denise Ottosen, and Rose Sawkins.

Great friends continued to cheer me on even as months of all-consuming writing stretched into years of declined invitations. Your enthusiasm means so much! Thanks particularly to Fran Freimarck, Michele Garrigan, Nancy Hein, Gary Pitts, and Helen Tait for volunteering to serve as beta readers.

A picture is worth a thousand words. Thanks to Jennifer Stimson for designing a cover that captures the spirit of *Eight Intentions* so beautifully.

Knowledge is an invaluable gift. Although this book bloomed from my personal experience, the wisdom shared by other authors provided the sunlight. Thanks to Stephen Covey, Louise Hay, David Hawkins, Esther and Jerry Hicks, Lynne McTaggart, Donna Eden, David Feinstein, Peta Stapleton, Clint Ober, Bruce Lipton, and Joe Dispenza.

ABOUT THE AUTHOR

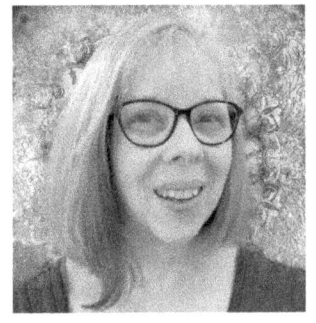

Drawing on her personal healing journey and coaching experience, Carolyn Pitts inspires others to maximize their health and self-healing capacity through informed lifestyle choices and energy medicine.

For over 25 years, Carolyn has maintained certification from the American Council on Exercise (ACE) as a Health Coach with specialization in behavior change.

A long-term proponent of the healing benefits of a whole food plant-based diet, Carolyn is certified through the Food Revolution Network as a Plant-Based Coach.

She is also a Healing Touch Professional with supplemental training in Healing Touch for Animals.

She has helped clients recover from surgery, chronic pain and insomnia, relieve the symptoms of autoimmune disease and cancer, as well as ease their end-of-life transition. Her experience with animals includes pets with chronic pain and behavior issues.

She is a member of the American College of Lifestyle Medicine, the Healing Touch Professional Association, and the HeartMath Institute, as well as a Power of Eight healing circle.

An avid believer in the healing power of the arts, Carolyn

serves on the Boards of local arts organizations. She regularly exhibits her high-vibe artwork in galleries and solo shows.

Carolyn shares wellness information on her YouTube channel, *Intend Well with Carolyn Pitts*, and through her newsletter, *The Intention Circle*.

Visit **CarolynPitts.com** to learn more.

youtube.com/@intendwell
linkedin.com/in/carolyn-pitts
goodreads.com/Carolyn_Pitts

www.ingramcontent.com/pod-product-compliance
Lightning Source LLC
Chambersburg PA
CBHW020535030426
42337CB00013B/861